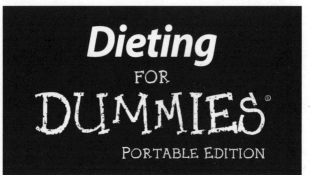

Dieting
FOR
DUMMIES®
PORTABLE EDITION

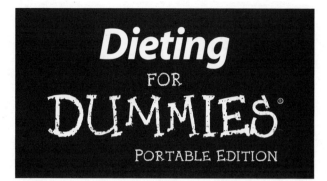

Dieting FOR DUMMIES®

PORTABLE EDITION

by Jane Kirby, RD
The American Dietetic Association

Core Strength For Dummies
excerpt by LaReine Chabut

WILEY

Wiley Publishing, Inc.

Dieting For Dummies®, Portable Edition

Published by
Wiley Publishing, Inc.
111 River St.
Hoboken, NJ 07030-5774
www.wiley.com

Copyright © 2009 by Wiley Publishing, Inc., Indianapolis, Indiana

Published by Wiley Publishing, Inc., Indianapolis, Indiana

Published simultaneously in Canada

For general information on our other products and services, please contact our Customer Care Department within the U.S. at 800-762-2974, outside the U.S. at 317-572-3993, or fax 317-572-4002.

For technical support, please visit www.wiley.com/techsupport.

Wiley also publishes its books in a variety of electronic formats. Some content that appears in print may not be available in electronic books.

ISBN: 978-0-470-44873-1

Manufactured in the United States of America

10 9 8 7 6 5 4 3 2 1

Publisher's Acknowledgments

We're proud of this book; please send us your comments through our Dummies Online Registration Form located at www.dummies.com/register.

Some of the people who helped bring this book to market include the following:

Acquisitions, Editorial, and Media Development

Project Editor: Elizabeth Kuball

Acquisitions Editors: Mike Lewis, Lindsay Lefevere

Copy Editor: Vicki Adang

Assistant Editor: Erin Calligan Mooney

Technical Editors: Kathryn Brown, EdD, RD, LD; Helen M. Seagle, MS, RD; Vicki I. Walker, MPH, RD; Damon Faust

Editorial Manager: Jennifer Ehrlich

Editorial Supervisor and Reprint Editor: Carmen Krikorian

Editorial Assistants: Joe Niesen, David Lutton, Jennette ElNaggar

Composition Services

Project Coordinator: Kristie Rees

Layout and Graphics: Kathie Rickard

Proofreaders: Laura Albert, Melissa Bronnenberg

Publishing and Editorial for Consumer Dummies

Diane Graves Steele, Vice President and Publisher, Consumer Dummies

Joyce Pepple, Acquisitions Director, Consumer Dummies

Kristin Ferguson-Wagstaffe, Product Development Director, Consumer Dummies

Ensley Eikenburg, Associate Publisher, Travel

Kelly Regan, Editorial Director, Travel

Publishing for Technology Dummies

Andy Cummings, Vice President and Publisher, Dummies Technology/General User

Composition Services

Gerry Fahey, Vice President of Production Services

Debbie Stailey, Director of Composition Services

Table of Contents

Introduction

● ●

Does the world really need another book on dieting? More important, do you? Plenty of diet books make promises that this one doesn't. Lots tell you that losing weight and keeping it off is easy and effortless when you know their secrets. Well, we have a secret to tell you that the other books won't: Dieting gimmicks, such as banning pasta, don't work. And that's precisely why you need this book. It's not about fad plans or take-it-off-quick schemes. It's about balancing healthful eating and exercise for a lifetime.

Another so-called *secret* that the other books don't tell you is that when you know the facts about how the exercise you do and the foods you eat regulate your weight, you can drop pounds and keep them off without ever eating another grapefruit — unless you like grapefruit, of course. We believe that knowledge is power: the power to *choose* to lose. That's what this book is all about.

You Can Trust Us

We know about losing weight, and this is what we bring to the table:

The American Dietetic Association is the largest organization of food and nutrition professionals in the world, with nearly 70,000 members. In other words, you can look to us for the most scientifically sound food and nutrition information available. Our members, with their extensive educational background, apply their knowledge of food, nutrition, culinary arts, physiology, biochemistry, anatomy, and psychology to help you translate nutrition recommendations into practical, clear, and straightforward advice.

We can't offer you a magic bullet to melt your extra pounds away, but we *can* provide a weight-loss and exercise plan that's realistic enough to last a lifetime. Since 1917, we have been serving the public through the promotion of optimal nutrition, health, and well-being by emphasizing a diet that includes variety, balance, moderation, and *taste*.

Jane Kirby is a registered dietitian and a member of the ADA. She is the food and nutrition editor of *Real Simple* magazine. She was the nutrition editor at *Glamour* magazine for 15 years and the editor-in-chief of *Eating Well* magazine. She's interviewed Doctors Ornish, Sears, Pritikin, and Atkins over the years. And she confesses to having been on all their diets — plus others. As Jane puts it:

You name it; I've tried it. I went on my first diet when I was about 12 years old; I drank Metracal (the 1960s version of Slim-Fast). By the time I got to college, I had a borderline case of anorexia nervosa. I dieted down to 98 pounds. (I'm 5'5".) I weighed as much as 160 pounds after my son was born (and that was *after* the birth). I've gained and lost about 250 pounds over my 50 years and spent about 30 years on the dieting treadmill. But I haven't dieted since my son was weaned 11 years ago. Today, I weigh 135. I know that I will never weigh 118 pounds (the weight that I always thought would make me smarter, prettier, richer, and happier). I don't starve myself, obsess about calories, or berate myself when I "fall off the wagon." But my cholesterol level is well under the 200 cutoff, and my HDL level (that's the good cholesterol) puts me at extremely low risk for heart disease. I don't eat everything I want to whenever I want it. (I do eat carefully.) I walk for at least one hour over the course of a day. I no longer believe that what I called my ideal weight is reasonable or attainable. Feeling great, and therefore looking great, is the goal. And it's comforting to read the new research that supports what my personal experience has taught me.

About This Book

Our experience as food and nutrition professionals (and former dieters) shows us that the key to successful weight loss doesn't require magic, grit and determination, or the moral character of a saint. Weight loss success also doesn't require that you read this book cover to cover. Chapters 1 and 2 can help you set reasonable goals and expectations. From there, though, feel free to skip around to chapters or topics that are of particular interest to you.

Some of the text topics may be familiar to you if you regularly read health magazines. This book aims to appeal to people whose nutrition knowledge ranges from shallow to deep. So if you're looking to dive headfirst into the subject, you won't be disappointed. And if you just want to get your feet wet, you can do that, too.

What You're Not to Read

Don't feel obliged to read every paragraph. Technical information, marked with a Technical Stuff icon, can enrich your understanding but it's not critical to your understanding or weight-loss success. The sidebars (boxes of text shaded in gray) function the same way — they're skippable. We hope you won't skip them, but know that the crux of the subject matter is in the running text.

Foolish Assumptions

This book is written for anyone who has eaten too much and wants to lose weight. The information presented here is appropriate for someone wanting to lose 10 pounds or 100 pounds. In fact, we hope you'll use it as a guide to eating healthfully, and not only a way to lose weight. Because, when you discover how to eat the healthy way, you *will* lose weight.

Icons Used in This Book

We include icons in the margins of this book to help you find the information that you're looking for more quickly. The following is a list of the icons and what they mean:

 This icon points to a tip that can make the dieting process easier.

 When you see this icon, you know that you're getting an important piece of information that's worth remembering.

 This icon warns you of dieting myths and dangers. Be wary!

 Because the dieting industry perpetuates many falsehoods, we use this icon to point out information that you can count on — and some fun facts, too.

 When we get a little technical and talk about scientific research, we use this icon. You can skip this stuff if it seems too far over your head, but it's good to know.

This icon demystifies the diet lingo that you so often hear. Find out what these terms mean, and you'll sound like a pro in no time.

Where to Go from Here

People come in a wide range of heights, weights, and girths. One is not better than another. But staying within *your* healthiest weight range can help you achieve optimal health and well-being. Join us in this book, starting at whatever point you like, and you'll see through the fog of fads and myths. Read on and find out how to stop dieting and start living healthfully.

Chapter 1

Getting Started

In This Chapter

▶ Understanding how weight affects health

▶ Tailoring a diet to suit you

▶ Recognizing the particulars

The first edition of *Dieting For Dummies* was published in 1999. Since then, however, the number of people who need to lose weight has exploded faster than a tub of popcorn at the cineplex. The science of weight loss has grown as well. We now have a better understanding of how our bodies store fat, how hunger is controlled, and why some people gain weight more easily than others. And we know more about applying the technical knowledge into practical how-to steps to help you lose weight and keep it off. That's what this book is all about. Translating the science of weight loss into an actionable weight-loss program that you can use.

Weighing In on Your Health

The statistics from the Centers for Disease Control are startling: Sixty-four percent of adult Americans are overweight or obese. It's a historic high — and it's scary when you realize that death as a result of being obese is closing in fast on the death rates from smoking. We start this book with health, because we think it's the most important reason to lose weight. It takes the emphasis off short-term goals — the vacation to the beach, for example — that promote the use of fad diets and gimmicks.

And, while we're on the subject, we should mention that we hate the idea of "going on a diet," because it means, eventually, going *off* the diet. But more important, diets are about denial. Humans are programmed for pleasure. We're wired to enjoy plenty of flavors and textures. Denying any one of the sensory aspects of food means that you'll eventually go off the diet.

The external messages and signals that bombard you are designed to make you eat, eat, eat. Unfortunately, those messages aren't about eating healthy foods. Portions are huge at restaurants; the ingredients and cooking methods that most affordable restaurants use and the items they serve all conspire against your health. Chapters 5 and 6 discuss in detail the ways you can spot the healthiest foods (in grocery stores and at restaurants) amid a tsunami of marketing terms, techniques, and tricks.

Getting motivated

Have you promised yourself that you'll get back to your senior-year weight before your 25th reunion? Or maybe you've vowed to lose weight before your wedding or your daughter's wedding. Everyone has set deadlines. And, unfortunately, most everyone has busted them. Losing weight to look better is one place to find your incentive. Many successful dieters get started with external motivators like appearance. Then as they progress on their weight-loss plan and start feeling healthier, their motivation internalizes.

When you start moving, not only will you start losing weight, but also you'll sleep better, be in a better mood, and have more energy than you've had in years.

Finding support

As you read through this book, you'll come across references to many studies that we've included to illustrate and support the ideas we're giving you. Most of them involve *successful losers* — people who lost weight and kept it off. We think that hearing their experiences can help you reach your goals, too. If we didn't think that the information in this book could help you to reach your goals, we wouldn't have written it. We may not have met face to face, but please know that we're rooting for you.

Setting goals

To figure out where you're headed, you need to know where you are. Chapter 2 can help you to examine your current weight and help you determine your healthiest weight — you may not have as much to lose as you think.

Understanding Conflicting Advice

"Eat pasta." "Don't eat pasta." "Diets don't work." "*This* diet does work." "Wine is good." "Alcohol can kill you." For every health claim, a counterclaim comes right back at ya. We understand that you're bombarded with information about eating right. In fact, if you rely on news reports to decipher nutrition advice, it may appear that recommendations change as often as a traffic light. Remember that news is news because it flies in the face of convention.

Despite the headlines, no one food or food group is better — or worse — than another. Folks today tend to remember the sound bite, not the big picture. This book gives you the big picture, because it's a summary of many studies, opinions, and recommendations and offers you the knowledge to understand the science.

One of the objectives of this book is to decipher and review all sides of the eating-advice controversy when conflicting opinions arise. For example, many well-respected scientists from well-respected research universities have heavily criticized the venerable Food Guide Pyramid. We explain the issues in Chapter 4 and tell you how the conflicting advice may affect how you eat.

Customizing Your Weight-Loss Plan

We promise you that this is the most personalized diet book you'll ever use, because it helps you write your own weight-loss plan. The weight-loss plan that you find in these pages is based on changing the ration of calories stored and calories burned. Of course, to lose weight you must burn more calories than you take in. (See Chapter 3 for more information.)

Obviously, one way to do that is to eat fewer calories. However, we don't want you to live your life counting calories and grams of fat or minutes of exercise. Of course, keeping lists and tallying calories is a good place to start. But eventually, your weight-loss plan will evolve into a healthy lifestyle. Eating for pleasure may sound like a frightening proposition if you're a typical overweight American. But when weight loss is about eating the things that *you* like and making your health a priority instead of an afterthought, success is assured.

You may have forgotten how it feels to be satisfied — rather than full or stuffed — after eating a meal. The goal is to turn down hunger and get back in touch with its subtle signals. That's part of eating nutritiously, too. Your body is wired to send codes and signals before, during, and after eating to tell you when to eat and when to stop. It's all part of Mother Nature's insurance that you survive. It's a remarkable system, but it's a little antiquated when you figure that (luckily) famine is rare in our society.

Eating is only half of a healthy weight-loss plan. We want to move you to move. We don't want to kid you into thinking that you can lose weight and keep it off without a little sweat. But you can incorporate exercise into your day without sucking yourself into a pair of spandex shorts or signing up for base-pounding Tae-Bo classes — unless you like that kind of thing, of course.

When an activity is fun, you're more likely to stick with it. The important thing is to find some form of exercise that you like to do.

Exercise not only improves your self-esteem, it helps the weight come off easily. It's yet another part of Mother Nature's grand scheme: Exercise burns calories, but it also regulates your appetite and keeps hunger in check.

Above all, just remember to think of this book as a reference. It's not just a book about dieting; it's a manual for healthy living.

Chapter 2

Assessing Your Own Weight

. . . .

In This Chapter

▶ Calculating your healthy weight range

▶ Determining your weight-related risk factors

▶ Getting pinched all over to calculate body fat

▶ Figuring out what all the measurements mean

. . . .

*W*hat exactly is a healthy weight? A healthy weight is a *range* that relates statistically to good health. Being overweight or obese is statistically related to weight-related health problems, such as heart disease and *hypertension* (high blood pressure). Health-care professionals use three key measurements to determine whether a person is at a healthy weight:

✔ **Body mass index (BMI):** A measure that correlates to how much fat is on your body.

✔ **Waist size:** A measure that helps to indicate whether the location of your body fat is a health hazard.

✔ **Risk factors for developing weight-related health problems:** For example, your cholesterol level, blood pressure, and family history.

What *you* should weigh for optimal health may be quite different from what someone else should weigh, even if that someone is your same height, gender, and age. The information in this chapter can help you determine what weight is best for you — your *healthy weight,* not the lowest weight that you think you can reach.

More than Just a Number

When you step onto your bathroom scale, the number shows you how much your total body weighs. This total includes fat, muscle, bone, and water. Even though a healthy weight depends on more than the number on the scale, that number is a general starting point that you can use to assess your weight.

When you know your weight, you can compare it to the healthy weight ranges of the *quick-estimate method* or use it to calculate your BMI (see the following sections). But what if your weight falls above these ranges? For most people, that's less healthy. The more that you weigh beyond and above the healthy weight range for your height, the greater your risk for weight-related health problems.

The information in this chapter is only for adults over 18 years old and should not be applied to children.

The quick-estimate method

To quickly estimate your healthy weight, you can use the following method. First, figure the median weight for your height by using the appropriate formula:

> ✔ **Men:** 106 pounds for 5 feet, plus 6 pounds per inch over 5 feet or minus 6 pounds per inch under 5 feet.

> ✔ **Women:** 100 pounds for 5 feet, plus 5 pounds per inch over 5 feet or minus 5 pounds per inch under 5 feet.

For example, if a man's height is 6', then his median weight is 178 pounds ($106 + [6 \times 12] = 178$). If a woman measures 5'5", then her median weight is 125 pounds ($100 + [5 \times 5] = 125$).

After you find your particular median weight number, you can calculate your healthy weight range. First, subtract 10 percent from your median weight (for the lower number in your healthy weight range) and then add 10 percent to your median weight (to find the higher number in your range).

Okay, go back to that 6' man. Ten percent of 178 pounds is about 18 pounds, so 178 pounds minus 18 is 160 pounds, and 178 pounds plus 18 pounds is 196. So the healthy weight range for a 6' man is between 160 and 196 pounds. As for the woman, who measures in at 5'5", we'll spare you the math and just give you the answer: Her healthy weight range is 113 to 137 pounds.

Body mass index

You can use body mass index (BMI) to determine whether you're at a healthy weight or overweight and, therefore, at a greater risk of developing weight-related health problems. BMI strongly correlates to the total fat on your body and, best of all, it's easy to determine and is applicable to all adults.

No more growing fat gracefully with age

For many years, weight charts were the only standards against which people compared themselves. Insurance companies, the publishers of these charts, emphasized an *ideal* weight as opposed to a *healthy* weight and held to different height and weight recommendations depending on age — one set of recommendations for ages 19 to 34 and another for ages 35 and older.

Later, the 1995 edition of Dietary Guidelines for Americans printed revised weight tables. An improvement over the age-based tables, the new tables indicated that a person's healthy weight range was the same regardless of age. Experts realized that the 10 to 15 pounds that many people put on as they age, although common, are not healthy.

Follow these steps to calculate your BMI:

1. **Convert your weight from pounds to kilograms.**

   Your weight (in pounds) ÷ 2.2 = your weight (in kilograms). For example, 132 pounds ÷ 2.2 kilograms = 60 kilograms.

2. **Convert your height from inches to meters.**

   Your height (in inches) ÷ 39.37 = your height (in meters). For example, 65 inches ÷ 39.37 meters = 1.65 meters.

3. Calculate your body mass index.

Your weight (in kilograms) ÷ (your height [in meters] × your height [in meters]) = BMI. For example, 60 kilograms ÷ (1.65 meters × 1.65 meters) = 22.03.

BMI is usually calculated in kilograms and meters, but if you feel more comfortable using pounds and feet, this formula will work for you: (your weight [in pounds] × 704.5) ÷ (your height [in inches] × your height [in inches]) = your BMI

 Table 2-1 enables you to determine your BMI without doing any math. Locate your height in inches in the left-hand column and follow the row across to your weight in pounds. Your BMI is at the top of the column at the intersection of your height and weight.

After calculating your BMI, you can determine whether you're at a healthy weight:

- ✔ **Healthy weight:** BMI of 19 to 24.9
- ✔ **Overweight:** BMI of 25 to 29.9
- ✔ **Obese:** BMI of 30 and above

BMI gives a more accurate assessment of body fat than weight alone, but it can overestimate body fat in people who are really muscular, such as linebackers or weightlifters, and it can underestimate fat in people who have lost plenty of muscle weight, such as your 100-year-old granny. And even if you have a normal BMI, you may not be at a healthy weight for you. Therefore, you also need to measure your waistline (see the following section).

Table 2-1   **Body Mass Index Chart**

BMI →	19	20	21	22	23	24	25	26	27	28	29	30	31	32	33	34	35	36	37	38	39	40	41
Height (inches)	**Body Weight (pounds)**																						
58	91	96	100	105	110	115	119	124	129	134	138	143	148	153	158	162	167	172	177	181	186	191	196
59	94	99	104	109	114	119	124	128	133	138	143	148	153	158	163	168	173	178	183	188	193	198	203
60	97	102	107	112	118	123	128	133	138	143	148	153	158	163	168	174	179	184	189	194	199	204	209
61	100	106	111	116	122	127	132	137	143	148	153	158	164	169	174	180	185	190	195	201	206	211	217
62	104	109	115	120	126	131	136	142	147	153	158	164	169	175	180	186	191	196	202	207	213	218	224
63	107	113	118	124	130	135	141	146	152	158	163	169	175	180	186	191	197	203	208	214	220	225	231
64	110	116	122	128	134	140	145	151	157	163	169	174	180	186	192	197	204	209	215	221	227	232	238
65	114	120	126	132	138	144	150	156	162	168	174	180	186	192	198	204	210	216	222	228	234	240	246
66	118	124	130	136	142	148	155	161	167	173	179	186	192	198	204	210	216	223	229	235	241	247	253

BMI →	19	20	21	22	23	24	25	26	27	28	29	30	31	32	33	34	35	36	37	38	39	40	41
Height (inches)	**Body Weight (pounds)**																						
67	121	127	134	140	146	153	159	166	172	178	185	191	198	204	211	217	223	230	236	242	249	255	261
68	125	131	138	144	151	158	164	171	177	184	190	197	203	210	216	223	230	236	243	249	256	262	269
69	128	135	142	149	155	162	169	176	182	189	196	203	209	216	223	230	236	243	250	257	263	270	277
70	132	139	146	153	160	167	174	181	188	195	202	209	216	222	229	236	243	250	257	264	271	278	285
71	136	143	150	157	165	172	179	186	193	200	208	215	222	229	236	243	250	257	265	272	279	286	293
72	140	147	154	162	169	177	184	191	199	206	213	221	228	235	242	250	258	265	272	279	287	294	302
73	144	151	159	166	174	182	189	197	204	212	219	227	235	242	250	257	265	272	280	288	295	302	310
74	148	155	163	171	179	186	194	202	210	218	225	233	241	249	256	264	272	280	287	295	303	311	319
75	152	160	168	176	184	192	200	208	216	224	232	240	248	256	264	272	279	287	295	303	311	319	327
76	156	164	172	180	189	197	205	213	221	230	238	246	254	263	271	279	287	295	304	312	320	328	336

Waist circumference

Even if you've never stepped on a scale or measured your height, you can use your waist measurement as an indicator of your health status.

You can't use your waist size to get an absolute percentage of body fat, but it does provide information regarding the *location* of your body fat. And knowing where your fat is located, along with your BMI, enables you to determine whether you're overweight and therefore need to lose weight.

Fat that accumulates around your stomach area makes you more susceptible to a variety of health problems. People who accumulate fat around their waists (known as *apples*) are at greater risk for developing serious chronic illness than are people who collect fat on their hips and buttocks, known as *pears*.

Follow these steps to get your waist circumference:

1. **Relax your shoulders and stand naturally.**

2. **With a tape measure, measure your waist at the point below your rib cage but above your belly button.**

   Make sure the tape is snug but doesn't pinch your skin and is parallel to the floor.

3. **Breathe out.**

4. **Read the number.**

If your BMI is 25 to 34.9 and your waist size is more than 40 inches if you're a man or more than 35 inches if you're a woman, you're at an increased risk of developing serious weight-related health problems. Even if your BMI falls into the healthy weight range of 19 to 25, you're at a greater health risk if your waist size is larger than your hips. Table 2-2 illustrates how waist circumference coupled with BMI increases your health risk for diabetes, high blood pressure, and heart disease.

Table 2-2	Health Risk of High Waist Circumference	
BMI	**Less Than 40 Inches Men/ Less Than 35 Inches Women**	**More Than 40 Inches Men/ More Than 35 Inches Women**
25.0–29.9	Increased	High
30.0–34.9	High	Very high
35.0–39.9	Very high	Very high
40.0 or above	Extremely high	Extremely high

Factoring In Your Personal Risk

You may decide to lose weight based solely on the size of your waist or by comparing your BMI to the BMI chart. But health-care professionals use more than these measurements to analyze your weight. They also look at weight-related risk factors before determining whether your weight is healthy.

The risk factors that health-care professionals look for include

- ✔ Age (older than 45 years old for males or 55 [or postmenopausal] for females)

- ✔ Arthritis in the knees or hips

- ✔ Family medical history of weight-related health problems

- ✔ Family history of early death (younger than 55 for males and 65 for females) from heart disease

- ✔ High blood pressure

✔ High blood cholesterol

✔ High blood sugar

✔ Respiratory problems

✔ Smoking

If you have any of the risk factors that I mention in the preceding list, even if you're in the healthy weight range, many health-care professionals may suggest that you lose 5 to 10 percent of your body weight to improve or lessen these risk factors. If you're over-weight, getting to your healthy weight is all the more urgent.

Do not even think about losing weight if you're pregnant or breast-feeding or less than 18 years old.

Using the Latest High-Tech Methods

BMI and waist size allow you to quickly compare your weight to the healthy weight range for your height and judge your relative "fatness." But other, high-tech ways are available to determine how much fat you have, which is often referred to as your *percent body fat*.

You may read about these methods in magazine arti-cles and weight-loss books or see that health clubs, commercial weight-loss programs, or even local uni-versity research facilities are offering them. But you should know that they're not the methods of choice because of impracticality or impreciseness issues. So keep reading to take a closer look at these various methods and their limitations.

Underwater weighing

Underwater weighing is the most accurate method for determining your percent body fat, but it's the least practical, because it's done with sophisticated equipment at university research facilities. This method is based on the premise that fat floats — think of how oil rises to the top in a bottle of salad dressing. Therefore, you can determine how much of your body is lean and how much is not if you submerge your body in a large tub of water.

To determine your percent body fat in this manner, you sit in a large tank or tub full of water in a special chair with a weight belt around your waist. (If you're thinking that this sounds more like a job for an escape artist cut from the same cloth as Houdini, try another method, because it gets worse — keep reading.) A trained technician then submerges you beneath the surface of the water as you force all the air out of your lungs. You must remain underwater for about 10 seconds so that the technician can record your weight. The technician repeats this procedure eight to ten times to determine an average. (See what we mean?)

To measure your body's volume, the technician computes the difference between your body's weight measured in air and its weight underwater. The technician then calculates your body density by dividing your body mass by the volume of the water that it displaces, minus any air left in your lungs. After computing density, the technician uses another formula to determine your percent body fat.

Skin-fold thickness

You've probably reacted negatively to being pinched in the past. It's not a nice thing to do to someone. But put your preconceived notions away for now and open up that mind of yours, because measuring *skin-fold thickness* (the amount of fat just under the skin) is a simpler method for determining percent body fat. When an experienced practitioner does the measuring, it's an accurate calculation of total body fat.

This method can yield inaccurate results if a less-than-skilled individual takes the measurements or if performed on an older person or on someone who is severely overweight. Given that the results can vary greatly depending on the practitioner, you should view the results skeptically.

To find out your percent body fat using the skin-fold test, a person trained to take a skin-fold measurement, such as a doctor, dietitian, or health-club staffer, measures your skin-fold thickness using skin-fold calipers at the upper arm, upper back, lower back, stomach, and upper thigh. The technician takes two sets of measurements and obtains an average at each site. Then he converts the millimeters that the calipers measure and places those numbers in a formula to arrive at the percent body fat of your entire body.

Now you know where the expression "pinch an inch" comes from. It may not be scientifically precise, but if you can pinch a 1-inch-thick (or more) fold of skin on the back of your upper arm, you're probably overfat.

Bioelectrical impedance

Okay, so the name *bioelectrical impedance* may sound like so much razzmatazz, but this method is legit and relatively easy to undergo. So quit rolling your peepers and keep reading.

Bioelectrical impedance is another relatively simple method for determining percent body fat, but it can produce inaccurate results if a person is dehydrated, overhydrated, severely overweight, or older with little muscle mass.

Assessing your weight based on percent body fat

If you ever have the opportunity to get your specific percent body fat measured by underwater weighing, skin-fold caliper, or bioelectrical impedance, use these estimated guidelines to assess your weight.

	Women	*Men*
Normal (optimal)	15 to 25 percent	10 to 20 percent
Overweight	25.1 to 29.9 percent	20.1 to 24.4 percent
Obese	30 percent or higher	25 percent or higher

Using bioelectrical impedance, a trained technician takes readings from a machine that delivers a harmless amount of electrical current through your body to estimate total body water, which reflects the amount of muscle or lean tissue you have. (Muscle contains water, and fat contains little water.) To determine the amount of body fat you have, the technician finds the difference between your body weight and your lean tissue.

Putting It All Together

Look back at your BMI, your waist size, and your percent body fat (if you have access to this measurement). Compare your numbers to the numbers in Table 2-3. Which column do you fit into?

Table 2-3		**Healthy Weight or Overweight?**	
		Healthy	*Overweight*
BMI		19 to 24.9	25 or higher
Percent body fat	Women	15 to 25	Over 25
	Men	10 to 20	Over 20
Waist size	Women	Varies	Over 35 inches (increased health risk when coupled with a BMI of over 25)
	Men	Varies	Over 40 inches (increased health risk when coupled with a BMI of over 25)

You probably don't need to lose weight if your weight is within the healthy range, if you've gained less than 10 pounds since you reached your adult height, and if you're otherwise healthy.

You *can* benefit from losing weight if you're overweight and you

- ✔ Carry excess body fat around your waist.

- ✔ Have weight-related risk factors.

- ✔ Have a family history of weight-related health problems.

If you're within a healthy weight range, your doctor may still suggest that you lose a few pounds if you have health problems (such as diabetes, high blood pressure, or arthritis) because of the increased risk.

The bottom line: Achieving and maintaining a healthy weight reduces your health risks. It also makes you feel better, increases your energy level, and boosts your confidence.

Chapter 3

Calorie Basics

. . . .

In This Chapter

▶ Measuring the energy in the food you eat

▶ Finding out about the big-kahuna calories

▶ Figuring out just how many calories you need

▶ Being honest about potential weight loss

. . . .

You eat calories. You count them. You shave them. You hate them. You've memorized the number of calories in your favorite foods. You know that eating too many calories makes you gain weight and that you lose weight when you eat fewer calories. But more than simply reading the numbers on food labels, calorie know-how means knowing *why* some foods have more calories than others and figuring out the number of calories that your body needs to survive and thrive are the first steps to getting started on a healthy weight-loss plan. This chapter explains all about calories and tells you how to manage them.

Defining Calories

 Although the technically correct name is *kilocalorie*, everyone, including dietitians, uses the shorter *calorie*.

Calories are simply a way to measure energy — the energy in food as well as the energy released in the body. Technically speaking, 1 calorie is the amount of energy necessary to raise the temperature of 1 gram of water by 1°C. You expend about 1 calorie per minute when sitting relaxed. That's about the same amount of heat released by a candle or a 75-watt light bulb.

Revealing Where Calories Come From

A calorie isn't a nutrient, but certain nutrients provide calories. Protein, carbohydrate, and fat make up the calorie contents of various foods. Although not considered a nutrient, alcohol also provides calories. In fact, one gram of

- ✔ **Protein** contains 4 calories.
- ✔ **Carbohydrate** contains 4 calories.
- ✔ **Fat** contains 9 calories.
- ✔ **Alcohol** contains 7 calories.

The remaining nutrients — water, minerals, and vitamins — do not provide calories, nor does fiber or cholesterol.

Few foods and beverages are 100 percent of any one nutrient. Most foods and beverages are a *combination* of protein, fat, and carbohydrate (and sometimes alcohol), so a food's calorie count is the sum of the calories provided by each nutrient. Here's how it works:

A bowl of chicken noodle soup contains 3 grams of protein, 7 grams of carbohydrate, and 2 grams of fat for a total of 58 calories:

3 grams protein × 4 calories/gram =
12 calories

7 grams carbohydrate × 4 calories/gram =
28 calories

2 grams fat × 9 calories/gram = 18 calories

Total = 58 calories

Even though most foods are made up of two or more
nutrients, foods are categorized by their predominant
nutrient. For example, a bagel and a bowl of cereal are
considered carbohydrate foods even though they also
contain protein and, sometimes, fat. Even though a
chicken breast is considered a protein food, not all of
its calories come from protein. Chicken also contains
fat, which contributes calories.

Not all calories are created equal. Foods that are
considered *empty-calorie foods* really have nothing in them as far as nutrition goes, except for
calories. Sugary foods, such as candy, are prime
examples. When you're restricting calories, you

Calorie counts

Calories are rounded on food labels, so when you multiply
the grams of protein, carbohydrate, or fat, you may come
out with a different value from what appears on the label.
Foods that contain 50 calories or fewer are rounded to the
nearest 5-calorie increment; foods with more than 50 calories are rounded to the nearest 10-calorie increment. And
foods that have fewer than 5 calories can be listed as
having 0 calories. Although you may think that this rounding
seems misleading or inaccurate, keep in mind that a 10-
calorie difference is actually negligible in the grand scheme
of things.

TECHNICAL STUFF

A burning issue: Measuring calories in food

Where do they get the calorie counts on food labels and in diet books? The old-fashioned way: They burn it.

The scientists who measure calories in foods call this method *direct calorimetry.* They use an instrument called a *bomb calorimeter,* essentially a highly insulated box containing a special oxygen-rich chamber surrounded by water. A food sample is placed inside the chamber and is burned completely. The heat released raises the temperature of the water in the box. How high the water temperature rises determines how many calories are in the food. If the temperature of the water increases by 10°C, for example, the food has 10 calories.

can make some room for empty-calorie foods but don't build your diet on them. If you do, you'll miss out on valuable minerals, fiber, and vitamins.

The opposite of empty-calorie foods are *nutrient-dense foods.* Calorie for calorie, they pack a solid nutrition punch by providing a good amount of vitamins, minerals, and/or fiber in comparison to the number of calories they provide. In other words, you get a big nutrition bang for your caloric buck. An example of a nutrient-dense food is an orange. For a mere 60 calories, you get about 3 grams of fiber, 100 percent of your daily vitamin C requirement, and a good amount of folic acid, plus a spectrum of other micronutrients and phytochemicals, such as antioxidants.

Tracking How Many Calories You Eat

Unfortunately, a magic formula for figuring out how many calories you eat is unavailable as yet — you simply have to track it. If you're keeping a food journal (a good idea), dig it out now.

If you aren't keeping one, or you can't find it, you can catch up: Buy a small notebook and write down *everything* you eat for two days during the week and one weekend day — including that handful of M&M's, the dressing you put on your salad, and the pat of butter you put on your potato. Don't forget to include beverages, too. People tend to eat differently on weekends from the way they eat on weekdays, so including a Saturday or Sunday in your tracking is important.

Make sure, too, to accurately estimate the amount of each food that you eat. Studies show that most people grossly underestimate their portion sizes — and then they can't figure out why they don't lose weight on their "diets"! The problem, of course, is that most people just eat too much.

The best way to determine how much you're eating is to weigh and measure your food. Fill your plate with the typical amount of food that you eat and then use a measuring cup, spoon, or scale to determine your serving size. Most people find it easiest to write down what they ate immediately following each meal; otherwise, they tend to forget about the incidentals, such as the glass of wine or soda, or the butter on the bread, and the amounts.

At the end of each day, go back and record the calories for each food you ate by using food labels or a
book of calorie counts. (You can usually find pocket-
size calorie-count books in the grocery-store checkout
line — and more-expanded versions in bookstores —
that list hundreds of foods.) Then simply tally the
number of calories for each food based on the amount
you ate, and total up for the day. After your three-day
recording period, add the total calorie counts together
and divide by 3. This gives you the approximate
number of calories (give or take a few) that you eat on
average each day.

Determining How Many Calories You Need

After you figure out how many calories you typically
eat, the next step is to figure out how many calories
you actually _need._ Not surprising, many people eat
more calories than they truly need, resulting in excess
weight.

Taking key factors into account

Your calorie needs are unique to you and depend on a
number of factors, including your age, sex, metabolism, activity level, and body size. The following list
covers in greater detail the factors that affect your
calorie needs.

To get a quick idea of your total calorie needs,
multiply your current weight by 15 if you're
moderately active or by 13 if you're not.

✔ **Your age:** Calorie needs peak at about age 25
and then begin to decline by about 2 percent
every 10 years. So if you're 25 years old and

need 2,200 calories to maintain your weight, you'll need only 2,156 by the time you're 35; 2,113 at age 45; 2,071 at age 55; and so on. One of the reasons for the reduced need is that an aging body replaces muscle with fat, which (unfortunately) burns fewer calories than muscle does. Yet, staying active and doing muscle-strengthening exercises keeps muscle mass intact. And even recent work with seniors proves that you can build muscle at any age.

✔ **Your sex:** An adult man has less body fat and about 10 to 20 percent more muscle than a woman of the same size and age. Because muscle burns more calories than fat does, a man's calorie needs are generally about 5 to 10 percent higher than a woman's.

Remember: The exception for women is during pregnancy and breast-feeding. During these times in your life, you definitely should *not* cut calories. In fact, you need to eat *more* calories — an extra 300 calories a day while pregnant and an extra 500 calories a day when breast-feeding.

If you're overweight when you become pregnant, talk with your doctor about an appropriate calorie level for you. Contrary to the old adage, pregnancy is *not* an excuse to eat for two (or three or more!), but you do need to be sure that you're taking in an adequate number of calories. The same goes for while you're breast-feeding.

✔ **Your metabolism:** A living body needs a minimum number of calories to maintain vital functions, such as breathing and keeping the heart beating. This minimum number is called basal metabolic rate (BMR). It's what most people are referring to when they talk about metabolism.

You can compare your body to a car's engine: Some run efficiently, and others take plenty of fuel to keep them moving. Researchers can predict BMR accurately by conducting a special test that measures how much oxygen the body uses within a set amount of time.

A quick and easy way to approximate your BMR without checking into a laboratory is to multiply your current weight by 10 if you're a woman or by 11 if you're a man. Your body needs about 10 to 11 calories, depending on your sex, for every pound you weigh to meet its basic needs. Therefore, a 150-pound woman needs about 1,500 calories a day; a 175-pound man needs about 1,925 calories. Additional calories are needed for digestion and activity. However, be aware that the more you weigh, the higher your calorie need will *appear* to be. You can find another, more accurate, way to determine your BMR that factors in your age in Table 3-1.

Table 3-1 How Many Calories Your Body Needs Per Day for Basic Energy Needs

Age	Use This Equation to Calculate Your BMR
Men	
18 to 30	$(15.3 \times$ weight [in kilograms]$) + 679$
30 to 60	$(11.6 \times$ weight [in kilograms]$) + 879$
Older than 60	$(13.5 \times$ weight [in kilograms]$) + 487$
Women	
18 to 30	$(14.7 \times$ weight [in kilograms]$) + 496$
30 to 60	$(8.7 \times$ weight [in kilograms]$) + 829$
Older than 60	$(10.5 \times$ weight [in kilograms]$) + 596$

✔ **Your genetic blueprint:** The metabolic rate that you inherit from your family in part determines the number of calories that your body needs to function, and you can't change this factor. That's why your friend who is at the same height, weight, and activity level as you are may be able to eat more calories than you and never gain weight.

Metabolic diseases that tend to be inherited, specifically those that affect your thyroid, can cause you to burn calories very quickly or very slowly. Though not as common as some people think, a malfunctioning thyroid gland can sabotage your best weight-loss efforts. Your physician can perform tests to determine your thyroid function.

✔ **Your body shape and the shape you're in:** Your body shape and size affect the number of calories you need. Muscle burns more calories than body fat does. So if you're solid and have a greater proportion of muscle to fat, your metabolism is higher. Likewise, if you have more body fat and less muscle, your metabolism is lower, and you have a greater tendency to store fat than someone who is tall and thin.

Remember: If you're large, you burn more calories doing an activity than an average-size person of the same sex and age does. The more you weigh, the more calories your body uses. That's one reason that men, who are usually bigger and weigh more than women, need more calories.

✔ **Your activity level:** When you're active, you burn calories. And if you burn (or expend) more calories than you eat, you lose weight. The kind of exercise you choose, and how long and how intensely you do it, determines exactly how many calories you burn. Some types of activity even help your body burn calories after you stop exercising — an added bonus!

Exercise, particularly resistance training, is also important to help minimize muscle loss that naturally occurs as you get older and during weight loss.

Putting it all together

Determining your body's total energy needs takes a bit of math — so grab a calculator and go figure.

Don't let the prospect of a little math scare you away. This method is easier than, and almost as accurate, as checking into a research lab and submitting yourself to scientific scrutiny by a white-coated nerd with a clipboard and a stopwatch. And, if precision isn't your thing, flip to the end of this chapter for a shortcut version. It'll get you in the ballpark, but without a specifically assigned seat.

Follow these steps:

1. **Estimate your basic energy needs.**

   You can use one of two methods: Multiply your current weight (in pounds) by 10 if you're a woman or 11 if you're a man. Or refer to Table 3-1, which factors in your age in addition to your sex.

   Remember: In the formula, *weight* represents your weight in kilograms, so translate your weight into kilograms by dividing the number of pounds you weigh by 2.2.

   For example: Sue is a 45-year-old female who weighs 155 pounds. She calculates her BMR like this:

   155 pounds ÷ 2.2 = 70.45 kilograms

   70.45 kilograms × 8.7 = 612.92 calories

   612.92 calories + 829 calories = 1,441.92 calories

So Sue's BMR — or the number of calories that her body needs at complete rest to function — is roughly 1,442 calories.

If you figure Sue's BMR by using the shortcut method, her needs are about 1,550 (155 pounds × 10 = 1,550) — a bit higher than the full calculation, but still in the same ballpark.

2. **Determine your activity factor value.**

   How active are you? Find the description in Table 8-2 that best matches your lifestyle. If you have a desk job but fit in a dose of daily exercise (at least 30 minutes), consider yourself in the light or moderate category.

Table 3-2	How Active Are You?	
If, Throughout Most of Your Day, Your Activities Include	*Your Activity Level Is*	*Your Activity Factor Is*
Sitting or standing; driving; painting; doing laboratory work; sewing, ironing, or cooking; playing cards or a musical instrument; sleeping or lying down; reading; typing	Very light	0.2
Doing garage, electrical, carpentry, or restaurant work; house-cleaning; caring for children; playing golf; sailing; light exercise, such as walking, for no more than 2 miles	Light	0.3
Heavy gardening or housework, cycling, playing tennis, skiing, or dancing; very little sitting	Moderate	0.4

(continued)

Table 3-2 *(continued)*

If, Throughout Most of Your Day, Your Activities Include	Your Activity Level Is	Your Activity Factor Is
Heavy manual labor such as construction work or digging; playing sports such as basket-ball, football, or soccer; climbing	Heavy	0.5

3. **Multiply your basic energy needs by the activity factor value that you determined in Step 2.**

    Using Sue as an example, she multiplies her BMR of 1,442 by 0.3 because her activity level is light — running around after her kids, taking care of the house, and fitting in a 2-mile morning walk with her neighbors every other day.

    $1,442 \times 0.3 = 432.6$ calories

    Sue needs 432.6 calories for her activity level.

4. **Determine the number of calories that you need for digestion and absorption of nutrients.**

    Eating food actually burns calories. Digesting food and absorbing nutrients uses about 10 percent of your daily energy needs. Add together your BMR and activity calories and then multiply the total by 10 percent.

    The calculation for Sue's calorie needs for digestion and absorption looks like this:

    $(1,442$ calories $+ 432.6$ calories$) \times 0.10 = 187.5$ calories

5. **Total your calorie needs.**

Add together your BMR, activity, and digestion/
absorption calorie needs to get your total calorie
needs — that is, the number of calories that you
need to maintain your current weight.

**To maintain her current weight of 155 pounds,
Sue calculates her total calorie needs like this:
1,442 calories + 432.6 calories + 187.5 calories =
2,062 total calories.**

Setting a Reasonable Calorie Level for Weight Loss

To lose weight, you have to cut down on how much
you eat — but not too much. If you try to cut too
many calories, you may not lose any weight at all.
When you cut calories severely, your metabolic rate
slows to adjust to the lower calorie level. In addition,
you probably won't be able to stick to your plan for
very long, because you'll be hungry all the time. This
section can help you find the right balance of calories
for you.

Too much food isn't the only cause of obesity;
lack of exercise is also part of the formula. So
when you think about dieting, you need to rede-
fine your definition to mean cutting calories *and*
upping exercise.

Don't cut your calorie level drastically when
trying to lose weight; this strategy will backfire.
Your body is programmed to defend your usual
weight, so when calories are cut severely — to
fewer than 800 to 1,000 a day — your metabolic
rate adjusts to conserve the few calories you do

give your body. You won't lose weight any faster than if you allowed yourself to enjoy 1,200 to 1,500 a day. Fortunately, when you overeat occasionally, your metabolism speeds up to burn the extra calories, too — ever striving to maintain your normal weight.

Knowing how many calories to cut

Because there are 3,500 calories in a pound and 7 days in a week, you can cut your daily calorie intake by 500 to lose 1 pound a week (3,500 ÷ 7 = 500). To lose 1½ pounds, you need to cut 750 calories a day. A 2-pound-a-week loss means eliminating 1,000 calories a day. A faster rate of weight loss is generally associated with weight regain and yo-yo dieting. Remember the tortoise and the hare: Slow and steady wins the race.

Look at how these guidelines affect Mary's weight-loss plans. After determining how many calories she needs each day to maintain her present weight, she knows that her present calorie level is about 2,472 calories each day. To lose 1 pound per week, Mary needs to cut 500 calories a day, bringing her weight-loss calorie level to 1,972. To lose 1½ pounds a week, her new calorie level would be 1,722 (2,472 – 750 = 1,722). Attempting to lose 2 pounds per week means that Mary's calorie allotment would drop to 1,472 calories. This amount, while still safe, may be too low for Mary's personal needs.

Using the 20 percent rule

If you're not eating many calories now and a reduction of 500 to 750 calories per day would put your calorie intake below 800 to 1,000 a day and, therefore, put your metabolism into low gear, use the 20 percent rule. It's a healthier way to lose weight.

First, figure out the average number of calories you eat now. To do so, see "Tracking How Many Calories You Eat," earlier in this chapter.

After you determine the average number of calories you consume, simply subtract 20 percent. We'll use Maureen as an example. According to Maureen's food records, she eats about 1,800 calories a day and would like to lose 20 pounds. Her calculations are as follows:

1,800 calories × 0.20 = 360 calories

1,800 calories – 360 calories = 1,440 calories

If Maureen cuts her calorie consumption by about 360 calories to 1,440 calories, she can lose between ½ and ¾ pound a week — a healthy rate of loss that won't leave her starving. In about seven months, Maureen should reach her goal. Slow and steady — but she's more likely to keep it off than if she tried to lose it in half that time.

Chapter 4

Putting Healthful Eating Guidelines into Practice

● ●

In This Chapter

▶ Letting the Food Guide Pyramid guide you

▶ Checking out food groups and portions

▶ Charting the course for weight loss

▶ Planning low-calorie meals

● ●

*T*he U.S. Department of Agriculture (USDA) Food Guide Pyramid, although widely criticized and reworked by some health groups, is the main tool that we recommend to help plan your diet. In this chapter, we fill you in on the controversies and suggest how you can use this information to make your diet the healthiest it can be. Look for paragraphs marked with the FYI icon that highlight the topics and recommendations under debate.

Glimpsing the Food Guide Pyramid

The Food Guide Pyramid (shown in Figure 4-1) is considered the mother of all pyramids. The Vegetarian, Mediterranean, and Asian Pyramid among others were modeled after this one. It's flexible, practical, and visual, so no matter what your eating preferences are, you can make it fit your lifestyle.

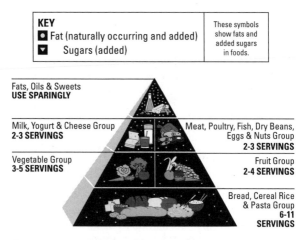

KEY	These symbols
◻ Fat (naturally occurring and added)	show fats and added sugars
▼ Sugars (added)	in foods.

Fats, Oils & Sweets
USE SPARINGLY

Milk, Yogurt & Cheese Group
2-3 SERVINGS

Meat, Poultry, Fish, Dry Beans, Eggs & Nuts Group
2-3 SERVINGS

Vegetable Group
3-5 SERVINGS

Fruit Group
2-4 SERVINGS

Bread, Cereal Rice & Pasta Group
6-11 SERVINGS

Figure 4-1: The Food Guide Pyramid helps you to put the Dietary Guidelines into practice.

The Food Guide Pyramid contains the building blocks for a healthy diet. If you follow the recommended servings listed for each food group in the pyramid each day and eat low-fat, low-sugar, and low-sodium choices within each group, you're sure to get enough protein, vitamins, minerals, and dietary fiber without getting excessive amounts of calories, fat, saturated fat, cholesterol, sodium, added sugars, or alcohol.

Notice that a range of servings is given for each block, or food group, of the pyramid. The serving sizes are designed to help people maintain their weights depending on how active they are. The lower number is intended to provide adequate nutrition for sedentary women, and the upper limit is for active teenage boys. Individuals who want to lose weight need to stick to the lower number of servings and sometimes go lower still.

 Hate the idea of counting calories? If you use the lower range of servings suggested in the pyramid, you'd be eating about 1,600 calories; the large number of servings totals 2,800 calories.

Fats and added sugars are concentrated in foods located at the tip of the pyramid. But they're also in foods found in the other food groups. When you choose foods for a healthy weight-loss diet, take the amount of fat and added sugars in those foods into consideration.

Remember:

- ✔ Choose low-fat foods from each of the food groups.
- ✔ Go easy on fats and sugars added to foods in cooking and at the table.
- ✔ Choose fewer foods that are high in sugars — candy, soft drinks, and sweet desserts.

Using the pyramid can help you identify where the bulk of your calories are coming from. Unfortunately, many people create a top-heavy pyramid by eating too much fat and sugar and not enough grains, fruits, and vegetables, as shown in the Actual Consumption Pyramid in Figure 4-2.

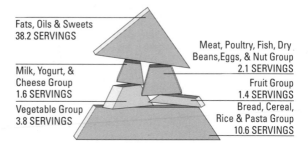

Fats, Oils & Sweets
38.2 SERVINGS

Meat, Poultry, Fish, Dry Beans, Eggs, & Nut Group
2.1 SERVINGS

Milk, Yogurt, & Cheese Group
1.6 SERVINGS

Fruit Group
1.4 SERVINGS

Vegetable Group
3.8 SERVINGS

Bread, Cereal, Rice & Pasta Group
10.6 SERVINGS

Figure 4-2: The Actual Consumption Pyramid.

Understanding What Makes a Serving

Of course, few people eat foods that fit neatly into one of the pyramid blocks. Pizza, for example, can be counted as dairy, grain, and depending on the topping, either meat or vegetables or both. A cheeseburger piled high with lettuce and tomato and a bit of mayonnaise counts as a serving from each group.

Table 4-1 lists the sizes of many foods that constitute one serving.

Table 4-1	What Counts as a Serving
Food Group	*One Serving Is . . .*
Bread, cereal, rice, and pasta	1 slice of bread; half a hamburger bun or English muffin; 1 small roll, biscuit, or muffin; 5 to 6 small or 3 to 4 large crackers; ½ cup cooked cereal, rice, or pasta; 1 ounce ready-to-eat cereal
Fruit	One whole fruit, such as a medium apple, banana, or orange; half a grapefruit; a melon wedge; ¾ cup fruit juice; ½ cup berries; ½ cup chopped fresh, cooked, or canned fruit; ¼ cup dried fruit
Vegetable	½ cup cooked vegetables; ½ cup chopped raw vegetables; 1 cup leafy raw vegetables, such as lettuce or spinach; ½ cup cooked beans, peas, or other legumes*; ¾ cup vegetable juice
Milk, yogurt, and cheese	1 cup milk, 8 ounces yogurt, 1½ ounces natural cheese, 2 ounces processed cheese
Meat, poultry, fish, dry beans, eggs, and nuts	Amounts should total 2 to 3 servings (for a total of 5 to 7 ounces) of cooked lean meat, poultry without skin, or fish per day. Count 1 egg; ½ cup cooked beans, peas, or other legumes*; or 2 tablespoons peanut butter as 1 ounce of meat.
Fats, oils, and sweets	Use sparingly.

* Note that you can count dry beans, peas, and other legumes as a serving of vegetables or a serving of meat, but the same bowl of beans can't count as a serving from both groups.

You've heard it before: It's not only *what* you eat but also *how much* that's important. As people eat more foods from restaurants and convenience stores, it's difficult to remember how large a serving should be. Portions of takeout food are huge — much larger than the standard portion sizes defined in the Food Guide Pyramid. Even cookbooks are instructing people to serve larger portions. For example, the 1964 edition of *The Joy of Cooking* recommends cutting a 13-x-9-inch pan of brownies into 30 bars; the 1997 version is cut into 16 bars.

A half-ounce of peanuts. An ounce of cheese. Two cups of popcorn. A quarter cup of sunflower seeds. A teaspoon of butter. A 3-ounce chicken breast. These are foods that you're apt to run into when you're eating on the run. After all, no one goes to a restaurant or movie theater packing measuring spoons or cups — at least no one we care to know. So how are you going to know what a serving of these foods look like?

A deck of cards is about the size of a 3-ounce chicken breast, but if the cards you play are on your computer screen more often than in your hand, you may not recognize what a portion looks like. But you take something with you wherever you go that can help you with portion size. It's in the palm of your hand. In fact, it *is* the palm of your hand, and it's the perfect portion measurement. That is, if you're an average female. Gentlemen, hold your honey's hand more often to get a sense of size. Better still, make sure to take her to restaurants and movies with you. Figure 4-3 gives you some other "handy" measurements.

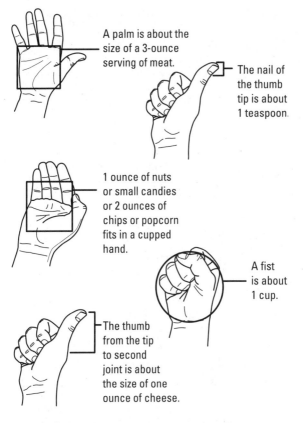

A palm is about the size of a 3-ounce serving of meat.

The nail of the thumb tip is about 1 teaspoon.

1 ounce of nuts or small candies or 2 ounces of chips or popcorn fits in a cupped hand.

A fist is about 1 cup.

The thumb from the tip to second joint is about the size of one ounce of cheese.

Figure 4-3: You can use your hand to judge portion sizes.

Looking at the Food Groups

All your favorite (and not-so-favorite) foods have a place on the Food Guide Pyramid. Foods are grouped together because their nutrient content is similar. And each of the five food groups, which we describe in detail in the following sections, supplies your body with some of the nutrients that you need for good health.

Some of the foods in the various groups may be higher in fat or added sugars than others, so when you're watching calories, focus on the lower-fat options that contain less added sugar.

The ground floor: Grains (6 to 11 servings)

Grains form the foundation of eating healthfully; they're low in fat and provide essential vitamins, minerals, and fiber. This group is the source of complex carbohydrates in your diet. But eating too many calories without getting beneficial nutrients is also common.

The grains group has been the source of the greatest controversy among health professionals. Critics think that too much emphasis is placed on carbohydrates as a foundation of a healthy diet and that the number of recommended servings is too high.

It's true that croissants, doughnuts, cookies, muffins, cake, and other high-fat and high-sugar items are in this group because they can fit into a healthy diet — just not everyday, and probably not more than once a week if you're trying to lose weight. Because they provide more calories than nutrients, keep them to a minimum. The healthier choice is anything whole grain in a reasonable portion.

Make sure that at least three of your grain servings each day are whole grains — whole-wheat bread or cereal, for example. Use the ingredient labels to find the products with whole grains: You want whole wheat or other whole grain to be the first ingredient. Sugar, oil, and fats should be last on the list, if they appear at all.

 Fiber comes from the grains group, the fruit and vegetable group, legumes in the meat group, and from nuts. Essentially, fiber is a carbohydrate that can't be digested. A healthy diet has 25 to 35 grams each day. High-fiber diets are associated with less heart disease and diabetes.

Second tier: Fruits (2 to 4 servings) and vegetables (3 to 5 servings)

Fruits and vegetables form the next layer of the pyramid. Both provide important vitamins, minerals, and fiber. Without high-fat toppings, such as butter and whipped cream, they're also naturally low in fat with few exceptions.

If you think that the number of servings of fruits and vegetables is impossible to consume each day, consider the fact that critics of the pyramid believe the recommendations are too low. For example, the Nurse's Health Study of more than 80,000 people demonstrated that people who ate more than eight servings a day had a 20 percent lower risk of heart disease than those who ate three or fewer servings. Further, their research showed that for each serving of fruits or vegetables, risk of heart disease decreased by 4 percent. Green leafy vegetables and vitamin C–rich fruits had the greatest effect.

Most of the news in nutrition research is about the
health benefits of a group of nutrients concentrated in
vegetables and fruits called *antioxidants*. These nutrients help minimize the normal wear and tear that
comes from living and can reduce the risk of cancer and
stroke as well as heart disease. Vitamins, such as *folate*
and *B6*, and the large family known as *carotinoids* —
such as *lycopene* in tomatoes, *beta carotene* in mangos
and carrots, *lutein* in spinach and collard greens, and
zeaxanthin in greens and corn — are some of the
antioxidants that have been identified. Yet researchers
point out that so many other phytonutrients that
haven't been isolated also factor in to the health benefits of eating more plant foods. Eating more fruits and
vegetables, instead of popping supplements, ensures
that you won't miss a single one.

Breakfast is a good place to begin building up fruit
servings. You may already start your day with a glass
of juice. Add a midmorning snack of fruit and have
some for dessert at lunch or dinner, and you've made
your goal of three to four servings a day.

Make at least one serving each day a citrus fruit.
Orange and grapefruit juice are standard options,
but don't forget about the many varieties of
oranges (navel, temple, Valencia, blood, and man-
darin) and grapefruits (Ruby Red, white, and
pink) that are available, as well as tangerines, tan-
gelos, kumquats, and Ugli fruit, which are also
considered citrus fruits. When possible, select
fresh fruit in season. In the Northern Hemisphere,
you can buy fresh strawberries in February and
apples in May. But because they aren't in season,
the fruit must be flown into the market from other
climates or put into storage. Out of season fruit
tends to be grown for longevity rather than flavor.
It's no wonder so many people are turned off by
fruit when it means red but flavorless winter
strawberries or mushy melons. Instead, choosing

oranges and grapefruit in winter and berries in spring, means there's a better chance that the fruit was grown locally and will end up tasting juicy and fresh.

Canned or frozen fruit can be a good substitute when a recipe or your appetite demands an out of season fruit. Be sure to reach for ones packed without added sugar.

Experiment with new fruits that you haven't tried before — figs, guava, star fruit, or prickly pears, for example. Many supermarkets stock large varieties of fruits worth investigating. Or you may want to use a meal out for a taste test, which can also give you an idea of an appropriate and skilled way to prepare the new fruits. Try less-common varieties of favorite fruits, such as Winesap or Rome apples; Casaba, Persian, or Santa Claus melons; or Comice or Seckel pears. Blend fresh or frozen fruits together with a dollop of low-fat yogurt, a splash of orange juice, and a ripe banana for a scrumptious fruit smoothie. Toss citrus segments, grape halves, or strawberries in with mixed greens and add low-fat poppy-seed dressing for a pretty and nutritious salad. Or sprinkle fresh or dried fruits on cereal, on frozen or regular yogurt, into muffin batter, or into rice and stuffing dishes.

With so many fruitfully delicious options to choose from, you'll never have to eat the same fruit twice in a week.

If it weren't for French-fried potatoes and tomato sauce on pizza and pasta, many people wouldn't get any vegetables at all. Too bad, because vegetables are mostly water, so they're a great way for dieters to expand their meals. Vegetables are a great source of vitamin C, folate, beta carotene, minerals, and fiber — and practically no fat.

Some vegetables are "starchy" and calorie dense; others are mostly water. If you're watching your weight, limit your starchy vegetables to one or two servings per day, and make the remainder of your veggie servings nonstarchy. Table 4-2 lists examples of starchy and nonstarchy vegetables.

Table 4-2	Vegetable Variations
Nonstarchy Vegetables	*Starchy Vegetables*
Asparagus	Beets
Broccoli	Cassava (yuca)
Brussels sprouts	Corn
Cabbage	Lima beans
Cauliflower	Peas
Celery	Potatoes
Chicory	Pumpkin
Cucumbers	Rutabaga
Eggplant	Sweet potatoes
Escarole	Taro
Green beans	Turnips
Greens (such as collard, kale, mustard, and turnip)	Winter squash
Lettuce	Yams
Mushrooms	
Okra	
Peppers	

Nonstarchy Vegetables	Starchy Vegetables
Radishes	
Sprouts	
Summer squash	
Tomatoes	

 Looking for ways to up your veggie intake? Try these delicious ideas:

✔ Pile a sandwich high with lettuce, tomato, and vegetables.

✔ Start every meal with a salad: a mix of dark green varieties of lettuce and colorful vegetables, drizzled with just a bit of low-calorie dressing.

✔ When you need a snack, reach for cherry tomatoes, celery, or sweet pepper strips. Many supermarkets carry small packages of celery or carrot sticks in their produce sections. They make good lunch-box (or briefcase) snacks for kids of all ages.

✔ Toss pasta with steamed broccoli, carrots, and other veggies and top with a smidgen of Parmesan cheese for pasta primavera. Or add finely chopped veggies — such as carrots, onions, cooked eggplant, squash, or chopped spinach — to pasta sauce.

✔ Toss a can of veggie or tomato juice into your briefcase for a quick pick-me-up (and a serving of vegetables to boot!).

✔ Top a baked potato with thick vegetable salsa or stir-fried vegetables.

Cruciferous vegetables

Cruciferous vegetables — bok choy, broccoli, Brussels sprouts, cabbage, cauliflower, kale, collards, kohlrabi, mustard greens, radishes, rutabaga, turnip, and watercress — are the cancer-fighters from the garden. They're called *cruciferous,* because their flowers or buds form a cross. Besides helping to protect against colon and rectal cancer, they're also good sources of calcium, iron, and folate.

Third tier: Meat and meat alternates (2 to 3 servings) and dairy products (2 to 3 servings)

Moving up the pyramid, you find foods that come mostly from animals — the Dairy group and the Meat, Poultry, Fish, Dry Beans, Eggs, and Nuts group. Foods from this level contribute important nutrients, such as protein, calcium, iron, and zinc.

Two to 3 ounces of meat, poultry, or fish (about the size of your palm) is an adequate amount of protein for a meal. Choose the select grades of beef, veal, and lamb to make sure that you get the least-marbled meats. Also, opt for lean cuts of meat, such as those from the round, loin, or leg (beef sirloin, ground round, or top round; pork tenderloin or loin chop; or leg of lamb). Select lean and extra-lean ground beef. Unless you're eating fat-free cold cuts, be extra cautious in the deli; many have more fat than lean meat per slice. Most fish are naturally lean.

 In the USDA view of the food world, meats, beans, nuts, and eggs are ganged together. They all do have higher amounts of protein than other foods in the pyramid, but that's where critics say the similarities end. Red meat has been associated with increased cancer risk, and some other meat, such as cold cuts, are particularly high in fat. New scientific evidence shows that nuts have vitamin E and beans have fiber that makes them more unique, not similar to meat. Plus, the fat in fish trumps the fat in red meat and chicken.

When meat is your protein of choice, trim all visible fat before cooking and remove the skin from poultry before eating. And use lower-fat cooking methods, such as roasting, broiling, and grilling instead of frying, sautéing, or pan-frying. Have fish a minimum of one day a week, and make at least one meal meatless. Dried beans and peas (legumes) are a good substitute for meat in this group.

The Milk, Yogurt, and Cheese group shares the third tier of the pyramid with the Meat, Poultry, Fish, Dry Beans, Eggs, and Nuts group. Like foods in the meat group, dairy foods are a good source of protein. They're also some of the best sources of calcium and contribute vitamins A and D to your diet as well.

A word of caution: Dairy foods can be very high in fat, so reach for fat-free, low-fat, part-skim, or reduced-fat cheeses, ice cream, frozen yogurt, ice milk, and fluid milk products when you're watching your weight. If dairy products aren't your cup of tea, so to speak, make sure you're getting enough calcium by eating more dark leafy greens. A supplement may also add to your daily requirement. But keep in mind that recent evidence shows that dairy products can actually help you lose weight. There have been many studies that prove it. One intriguing body of work done at the University of Tennessee and published in the medical journal *Lipids* in February 2002 concluded that increasing dietary sources of calcium, especially from dairy products, reduced body fat even without calorie restriction and accelerated weight loss when calories were cut.

If you're lactose intolerant and can't eat dairy products without becoming ill, consider milk that has been treated to reduce the amount of lactose in it. You can find several brands on the market that are worth a try.

 Don't mistake cheese for the only ideal protein alternative to meat. Sure it delivers some protein, but it also comes with an abundance of fat. If you choose not to eat meat from the meat group, go for water-packed tuna, bean and bean spreads, such as hummus (made with a minimal amount of tahini paste), and soy products, such as tempeh and tofu. Or choose reduced-fat cheeses or lower-fat varieties, such as feta, baby Swiss, and part-skim mozzarella.

Alcohol in your diet

Although alcohol isn't technically part of the pyramid, keep in mind that like items from the pyramid's tip, you get calories but no nutrients in each and every glass. Limit your consumption to no more than two drinks per day if you're male and one drink per day if you're female.

A serving of alcohol is defined as

- 12 ounces of beer

- 1½ ounces of hard or distilled spirits (80 proof)

- 5 ounces of wine

The tiny tier: Fats, oils, and sweets

Just because this group is on the top of the pyramid doesn't mean that it's the best group. Instead, this placement means that, like a penthouse, few people can spend much time there. Scan Table 4-3, and you'll see plenty of foods that you probably eat frequently. Most of these foods contribute practically no nutrients other than sugar, fat, and calories.

Grouping all fats with sugars riles some health groups. There's not much evidence to justify eating more sugar. However, critics say locking all fats and oils in the attic with sugar and sweets simply isn't fair. All fats have the same number of calories, but consider the bigger picture: Trans fats, found in foods made with partially hydrogenated fat, such as some stick margarines and solid vegetable shortening, are as unhealthy as *saturated fat* — animal fat that's solid at room temperature. Both raise unhealthy LDL cholesterol and contribute to heart disease. Unsaturated fats, on the other hand, improve cholesterol levels and thus lower heart disease risk. The oils of nuts, seeds, and olives are unsaturated. The bottom line: Use any fats sparingly — they're caloric — and when you do, make them unsaturated.

Table 4-3   Fats and Sugars — Use Sparingly!

Fats	Sugars
Bacon and salt pork	Candy
Butter	Corn syrup
Cream (dairy or nondairy)	Frosting (icing)

(continued)

Table 4-3 *(continued)*

Fats	Sugars
Cream cheese	Fruit drinks (unfortified)
Lard	Gelatin desserts
Margarine	Honey
Mayonnaise	Jam or jelly
Salad dressing	Maple syrup
Shortening	Marmalade
Sour cream	Molasses
Vegetable oil	Popsicles and ices
	Sherbet
	Soft drinks
	Sugar (white and brown)

Considering the Vegetarian Pyramid

If you don't eat meat, check out the Vegetarian Pyramid, shown in Figure 4-4. Because meat, poultry, and fish are not included in a vegetarian-eating plan, the foundation of this pyramid is divided equally among fruits and vegetables, legumes — such as soybeans and peanuts, and whole grains. Vegetarians should include foods from these three groups at every meal. Nuts and seeds, milk or soymilk, and oils should be consumed daily, and eggs and sugars only occasionally and in small quantities. But dieters should remember that servings of nuts, seeds, and oils should be small, because they're high in fat, and therefore, calories.

(c) ADAF 1997.

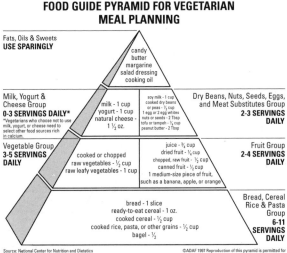

FOOD GUIDE PYRAMID FOR VEGETARIAN MEAL PLANNING

Fats, Oils & Sweets
USE SPARINGLY

candy
butter
margarine
salad dressing
cooking oil

Milk, Yogurt & Cheese Group
0-3 SERVINGS DAILY*
*Vegetarians who choose not to use milk, yogurt, or cheese need to select other food sources rich in calcium.

milk - 1 cup
yogurt - 1 cup
natural cheese - 1 ½ oz.

soy milk - 1 cup
cooked dry beans or peas - ½ cup
1 egg or 2 egg whites
nuts or seeds - 2 Tbsp
tofu or tempeh - ¼ cup
peanut butter - 2 Tbsp

Dry Beans, Nuts, Seeds, Eggs, and Meat Substitutes Group
2-3 SERVINGS DAILY

Vegetable Group
3-5 SERVINGS DAILY

cooked or chopped raw vegetables - ½ cup
raw leafy vegetables - 1 cup

juice - ¾ cup
dried fruit - ¼ cup
chopped, raw fruit - ½ cup
canned fruit - ½ cup
1 medium-size piece of fruit, such as a banana, apple, or orange

Fruit Group
2-4 SERVINGS DAILY

bread - 1 slice
ready-to-eat cereal - 1 oz.
cooked cereal - ½ cup
cooked rice, pasta, or other grains - ½ cup
bagel - ½

Bread, Cereal Rice & Pasta Group
6-11 SERVINGS DAILY

Source: National Center for Nutrition and Dietetics
The American Dietetic Association: Based on the USDA Food Guide Pyramid

©ADAF 1997 Reproduction of this pyramid is permitted for educational purposes. Reproduction for sales purposes is not permitted.

Figure 4-4: The Vegetarian Pyramid.

Using the Pyramid for Weight Loss

After you have a general idea of which foods belong in which food groups, you can start to plan your weight-loss diet. First, revisit the material in Chapter 3 to determine your calorie needs. Then, using the information in Table 4-4, determine the number of servings from each food group that you're allowed, based on your calorie level.

Table 4-4	Food Group Servings for Various Calorie Levels		
	About 1,200 calories	About 1,500 calories	About 1,800 calories
Bread group servings	5	6	8
Vegetable group servings	3	3	5
Fruit group servings	2	3	4
Milk group servings	2	2	2
Meat group	5 ounces	6 ounces	7 ounces
Fats, oils, and sweets	Use very sparingly	Use very sparingly	Use very sparingly

The Weight-Loss Pyramid, shown in Figure 4-5, is just like the Food Guide Pyramid, except that the number of servings from each group is decreased to the minimum amount needed for good health. When you're dieting and cutting calories, it's more important than ever to choose nutrient-dense foods and not waste calories on "extras" or high fat/sugar/calorie foods that provide little in the way of vitamins and minerals.

For the 1,200 calorie diet, you may notice that the number of bread servings allowed is five — less than the usual minimum of six servings for the traditional Food Guide Pyramid. But don't worry; cutting back on a serving of bread won't put you at a loss for nutrients. You get plenty of the B vitamins and fiber that your body needs from five servings. Just make sure that your choices from this group are whole grain and high in fiber.

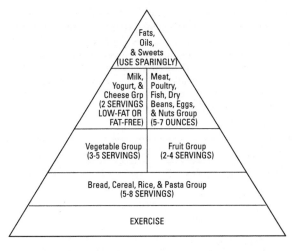

Figure 4-5: The Weight-Loss Pyramid.

It's also sometimes difficult to get the 1,000 to 1,200 milligrams of calcium required from just two servings of dairy. To help boost your calcium intake from other food sources, include a serving of dark green, leafy vegetables; drink a glass of calcium-fortified orange juice as one of your fruit servings; and, for health insurance, include a calcium supplement.

 Meeting all your nutrient requirements is difficult when drastically limiting calories. If your calorie intake is 1,200 calories or lower, be sure to take a multivitamin-mineral supplement.

Planning Your Meals

How do you keep all these portion sizes and food groups straight? A simple sheet of paper can help. Make a grid like the one shown in Table 4-5, placing the days of the week across the top and the food groups down the side. Next to each food group, write the number of servings that your calorie level allows. Then, each day, make Xs in the appropriate columns until you reach your daily allotment. Not only is this chart a quick visual reference for you, but studies show that dieters who track what they eat each day are more successful in losing weight and keeping it off.

Table 4-5	Sample Week at 1,200 Calories						
Food Group	*M*	*T*	*W*	*T*	*F*	*S*	*S*
Bread (5)	xxxxx						
Fruit (2)	xx						
Vegetable (3)	xx						
Meat (5 ounces)	xxx						
Milk (2)	xx						
Fats, oils, and sweets	x						

If you see that you've had all your meat and dairy for the day, for example, and you want something to snack on, try a piece of fruit or a few raw vegetables if you haven't had all your servings for the day.

A sample day may look like the following:

Breakfast:

- ✔ 6 ounces orange juice (fruit)
- ✔ 1 slice whole-wheat toast (bread)

✔ Hard-cooked egg (meat)

✔ Jelly (fats, oils, and sweets)

> **TIP** Don't skip breakfast. Your mother was right, and so are the 3,000 people in the National Weight Control Registry (NWCR). These people are losers! As in, on average each lost about 60 pounds and kept it off for about 6 years. A 2002 study in the journal *Obesity Research* reported that only 114 of the 3,000 didn't eat breakfast.

Lunch:

✔ Turkey sandwich made with 2 ounces of meat (2 bread, 2 meat)

✔ Lettuce and tomato (vegetable)

✔ 1 cup fat-free milk (milk)

✔ One-quarter cantaloupe (fruit)

Snack:

✔ 2 cups popcorn (bread)

✔ Diet soda (free)

Dinner:

✔ 2 ounces of broiled fish (meat)

✔ 1 small baked potato (vegetable)

✔ ½ cup broccoli (vegetable)

Snack:

✔ Apple (fruit)

✔ 1½ ounces low-fat cheese (dairy)

✔ 5 saltine crackers (grain)

"Free" foods may not be so free

Certain foods are considered "free" foods, because they provide almost no calories. Examples of free foods include sugar-free hard candies or chewing gum, diet soft drinks or drink mixes, club soda, sugar-free gelatin, and bouillon or broth. Using these free foods as extras throughout the day is fine, but don't overdo them. Although each one individually provides few calories, if you go overboard with some of them, the sodium can start to add up.

Tailoring Your Diet to Include Healthier Choices

To plan your diet, you can follow a printed diet sheet that offers no choice or variation regardless of your personal taste preferences. But what happens when you reach your goal weight? What have you discovered? Better to use the weight-loss process as a learning experience toward making healthier food choices. When you make those choices, keep these three points in mind.

Variety

You can achieve a healthful, nutritious eating pattern with many combinations of foods. For the best variety, choose foods within and across food groups, because foods within the same group have different combinations of nutrients and other beneficial substances. For example, chicken, beef, pork, and fish all contain iron, but in varying amounts; pork has more B vitamins than other protein choices. Some vegetables and fruits are good sources of vitamin C or vitamin A,

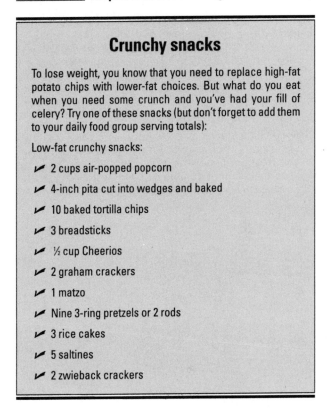

Crunchy snacks

To lose weight, you know that you need to replace high-fat potato chips with lower-fat choices. But what do you eat when you need some crunch and you've had your fill of celery? Try one of these snacks (but don't forget to add them to your daily food group serving totals):

Low-fat crunchy snacks:

- ✔ 2 cups air-popped popcorn
- ✔ 4-inch pita cut into wedges and baked
- ✔ 10 baked tortilla chips
- ✔ 3 breadsticks
- ✔ ½ cup Cheerios
- ✔ 2 graham crackers
- ✔ 1 matzo
- ✔ Nine 3-ring pretzels or 2 rods
- ✔ 3 rice cakes
- ✔ 5 saltines
- ✔ 2 zwieback crackers

and others are high in folate; still others are good sources of calcium or iron. Choosing a variety of foods within each group also makes your meals more interesting from day to day.

Balance

You need to balance the kinds and amounts of food on your plate as well as what you eat over the course of a day and over an entire week. The most satisfying meals are a combination of protein foods, grains, vegetables, and fruits. A lunch of only salad or a breakfast of only a bagel and coffee won't stay with you for long. But if you build balance into your meals, you'll feel satisfied longer.

Moderation

Keeping portions moderate in size and content allows for flexibility. You may find room for a small or kiddie-size treat even on a weight-reduction diet — but probably not a super-size treat.

Chapter 5

Healthy Grocery Shopping

More places sell food today than at any other time in history. Just five years ago, people bought gas at a gas station. Today, they can buy all kinds and sizes of snacks and sodas — and plenty of calories. If you don't plan ahead and do a weekly or twice-weekly grocery run, you may be forced to shop at the quick stop. That means being faced with aisles of foods that shout, "Buy me! Eat me!" It's a jungle of temptation out there. To stay on the weight-loss track, arm yourself with the tips in this chapter.

Making a Healthy Grocery List

Shoppers who use lists spend slightly more money per trip to the grocery store than nonlist users, but they don't have to run back to the market as frequently to pick up forgotten items. The benefit to dieters: Temptation has fewer chances.

 Some tips for making sure that your grocery list is diet friendly and that your trip to the store is as quick and painless as possible are as follows:

- **Plan your menus when you're hungry.** They'll be more interesting. But shop when you're not hungry, so you'll have more control.

- **Forget using coupons, unless they're for food items that you usually buy.** The savings can be tempting, but the purchase can add up to a diet disaster.

- **Check your cupboards, freezer, and refrigerator in advance to avoid duplicating purchases.**

- **Find out the store's layout and write your list according to it.** You'll be less likely to forget items. Or write your list according to categories: frozen foods, produce, meat, and dairy, for example.

Filling Your Grocery Cart the Right Way

Your menus, shopping list, and filled grocery cart should be in the same proportion as the Food Guide Pyramid: whole-grain bread, cereal, rice, and pasta should occupy the largest space and be the foundation on which the rest is built. Fruits and vegetables come next in order of predominance, followed by meat and dairy. Fats, oils, and sugar should take up the least amount of space. Keep reading for some specifics about the Food Guide Pyramid's recommendations.

Breads, cereals, rice, and pasta

Thick-sliced, thin-sliced, with sugar or without, whole-grain or white, this category has grown to one of the most confusing and calorie dense in the store. Shop carefully and heed these hints.

- ✔ **When you buy breads, make sure that the first grain on the ingredient list is a whole grain, such as whole wheat, oats, or millet.** Note that rye and pumpernickel breads aren't whole grain, even though their color may make you think that they are. Their fiber content is similar to that of white bread, but the calorie content is often slightly higher, because molasses is added for color.

- ✔ **Baked goods should have 3 grams of fat or less per serving.** And cereal should have at least 3 grams of fiber per serving.

- ✔ **Pizza dough or crusts should be whole wheat.** Search them out or ask your grocer to stock them.

- ✔ **Frozen waffles and pancakes should be low-fat.**

- ✔ **Baked goods from the in-store bakery don't usually have nutrient labeling.** Look at the ingredient list to see what kinds of flour are used. Go for the ones that list whole-grain flours first.

- ✔ **Avoid giant muffins, biscuits, and scones.** One has several servings' worth of fat and calories. One store-bought brand-name bran muffin has 160 calories and 7 grams of fat. Depending on the recipe, a homemade bran muffin may have much less. One muffin made per the recipe in the 1964 edition of *The Joy of Cooking*, for example, has 135 calories and 4 grams of fat.

✔ **When you read labels on packaged mixes, be sure to look at the "As Prepared" column.** Many mixes call for fats or eggs to be added in preparation.

✔ **Brown rice has almost three times the fiber of white rice.**

✔ **Ramen noodle soups are flash-cooked in oil before packaging, which means that they're high in fat.**

✔ **A sugar-sweetened cereal that has 8 grams of carbohydrate per serving has the same amount of sugar as an unsweetened cereal to which one rounded teaspoon of sugar has been added.**

✔ **Seeded crackers have slightly more calories than plain ones, but they have more fiber, too.**

Fruits and vegetables

No question about it: Fruits and vegetables are almost *free* foods for dieters. But eating healthfully means more than counting calories. Vitamins and minerals are important, too. Want to get more nutrition out of your fruits and vegetables? Follow these tips:

✔ **In general, the darker the color, the higher the nutrient content.** Dark salad greens, such as spinach, watercress, and arugula contain more nutrients than pale ones, such as iceberg lettuce. Deep orange– or red-fleshed fruit, such as mangoes, melon, papaya, and oranges, are richer in vitamins A and C than pears and bananas, but pears and bananas are especially good sources of potassium and fiber.

✔ **For the best buy and best flavor, get fresh fruits and vegetables while they're in season.** Otherwise, canned or frozen forms processed without added sugar, fats, or sauces are a good choice.

✔ **Fresh produce doesn't carry nutrient labels; look for nutrition flyers or posters in the produce department for specifics.** If prepared without sauces, butter, or added sugar, most fruits weigh in at less than 60 calories per ½ cup serving. Most vegetables contain a mere 25 calories per ½ cup cooked serving or per 1 cup raw.

✔ **Most fresh produce is virtually fat free, with the exception of avocado and coconut.**

✔ **Shop the salad bar when you need ingredients for a recipe, but don't purchase more than you can use at one time.** Cut ingredients will lose nutrients faster than whole. Cut produce in bags is packaged in special material that cuts down on moisture loss and, therefore, nutrient loss, too.

✔ **Prebagged salad is a staple in every supermarket.** Buy the salad that's packaged without dressing packets or garnishes. (These items are high in fat and calories.) And for a longer shelf life at home, buy bags of single-variety lettuces and create your own mix. Fragile leaves in salad blends can spoil quickly, ruining the whole bag.

✔ **Dried fruits are a healthy, high-fiber snack food, but because most of the water has been removed from them, the nutrients are concentrated and the calories are higher.** Keep an eye on serving size.

✔ **Many dried fruits, especially bananas, cranberries, and dates, have sugar added to them.**

Dairy

One of the first foods to be cut from many dieters' shopping lists and menus is dairy. What a shame! Most people, women in particular, need to *increase* their dairy consumption, because they don't get enough precious, bone-building calcium.

Plus, incorporating more dairy products can actually enhance weight loss according to accumulating research. In the February 2002 issue of *Lipids,* a medical journal, research at the University of Tennessee concluded that increasing dietary sources of calcium, especially from dairy products, reduces body fat, even without calorie restriction and accelerates weight loss when calories are reduced.

Low-fat dairy products are among the best-tasting fat-reduced items in the supermarket, and they have all the calcium of the full-fat varieties. Don't cut out dairy products altogether — just cut down on the high-fat (and high-calorie) dairy foods. Look for the following when you shop:

✔ **Buy only low-fat (1 percent) or fat-free (skim) milk.** Two-percent milk isn't low-fat. Low-fat or fat-free milk is often fortified with nonfat milk protein to improve its texture. An added bonus is that it has a bit more calcium than whole milk.

✔ **Buy only low-fat or nonfat yogurt and cottage cheese.** Creamed cottage cheese (4 percent milk fat) doesn't have cream added to it; it's made with whole milk. The name refers to the way it's processed.

✔ **Search out and buy low-fat cheeses.** They're labeled *part skim, reduced fat,* or *fat free.* However, strongly flavored, full-fat cheeses are fine if used sparingly.

✔ **Buttermilk contains no butter and is available in low-fat and fat-free varieties.** Some dieters find that its thicker texture is more satisfying than that of fat-free milk.

Meat, poultry, fish, dry beans, eggs, and nuts

Many dieters make the mistake of thinking that if they cut out meat, they cut out calories. Unfortunately, they often substitute high-fat cheese, nuts, and nut butters for protein. Without meat, getting enough zinc and iron — two nutrients that help maintain your energy and performance — is tough.

 Don't shortchange yourself nutritionally by making sacrifices that don't help. Shop smart instead. See the suggestions that follow:

- **Some of the leanest cuts of beef are flank, sirloin, and tenderloin.** The leanest pork is fresh, whole canned hams, cured, and boiled ham. Canadian bacon, pork tenderloin, rib chops, and roast are also on the lean side. Lean lamb includes roasts, chops, and legs; white-meat poultry is lower in fat than dark.

- **Meat labeled *select* is leaner than meat graded *choice*.**

- **Turkey or chicken skin is high in fat and calories.** When you shop, look for a label that reads ground turkey or chicken *meat* for the lowest fat. Or better yet, look for a label that reads *ground turkey breast,* which is lower still.

- **Self-basting turkeys have fat injected into the meat.** Dieters should avoid them.

- **Buy water-packed tuna and sardines rather than those packed in oil.**

- **Buy only fresh seafood or seafood that's frozen without added breading or frying.**

✔ **Cold cuts should be low-fat.** Turkey and chicken franks don't always have fewer calories than beef or pork; check the labels.

✔ **A half-cup of beans or 3 ounces of tofu equals a serving of protein.** Check the ingredient list for calcium sulfate. Tofu processed with it is a good source of calcium.

Better beef for your burger

When well done, the nutritional difference between a burger made with regular ground beef and one made with extra lean doesn't amount to much. When broiled on a rack or grilled, about 2 ounces of fat drips out of the regular meat. Lean meat loses a similar amount of weight, but it's fat plus water. A well-done burger made with 4 ounces of regular ground beef or chuck has only 12 calories more than a same-size, extra-lean burger, and has almost the same number of calories as one made with lean ground beef. The big difference is in price and flavor — regular ground beef or chuck wins on both counts.

Ground Beef	Raw		Cooked (Well Done)	
	Calories	Fat (Grams)	Calories	Fat (Grams)
Extra lean (17% fat)	264	19	186	11
Lean (21% fat)	298	23	196	12
Regular (chuck) (27% fat)	350	30	198	13

✔ **Two tablespoons of peanut butter counts nutritionally as an ounce of meat, but at 190 calories and 16 grams of fat, it's hardly a dieter's best bet.** Even reduced-fat peanut butter has 12 grams of fat, and because it has added sugar, the reduced-fat and regular versions have the same number of calories.

Fats, oils, and sweets

At the very top of the Food Guide Pyramid is the tiny triangle of fats and sweets. These foods add calories without contributing much in the way of other nutrients to your diet. Use them sparingly. But do remember that when you plan carefully, you can make room for these fun foods, too. Consider these tips:

✔ **With the exception of whipped or diet spreads, all butter, margarine, and oils have about 100 calories per tablespoon.** Whipped has about 70, and light varieties have 50 to 60.

✔ **Sugar, syrups (such as pancake and maple), and jelly beans don't add fat, but that doesn't mean that they're free foods.** They still have calories. One *level* teaspoon of sugar has 16 calories — surely not enough to ruin your diet, but if you have 3 cups of coffee and a bowl of cereal a day and use 2 teaspoons of sugar in each, that's a quick 128 calories. If you substituted no-calorie sweeteners for this amount of sugar and made no other changes in the way you ate, you'd lose 1 pound in a month.

✔ **Keep nuts on your shopping list, because they contain heart-healthy antioxidants and make great snack foods.** But buy them in the shell. Opening the shells as you eat will slow you down, so you don't wolf them by the fistful.

Navigating the Supermarket Maze

Supermarkets are sophisticated marketing systems. Everything you see and smell in a grocery store is specifically crafted to entice you to buy more. Where items are placed in the store, whether a package meets you at eye level or your child's eye level, the amount of time the aroma of chickens roasting in the deli wafts under your nose, the brightness of the lights, the tempo of the music — everything is carefully chosen.

To effectively navigate the supermarket maze, remember to

- **Double-check the end-of-aisle displays against the usual in-aisle stock.** The items featured at the ends of the aisles aren't always on special.

- **Eat before shopping and feed the children, too.** Hunger makes controlled shopping difficult for adults and nearly impossible for children.

- **Refuse to be tempted by free samples.** If you're not hungry, you're better able to pass them by.

- **Realize that the most frequently purchased foods are placed farthest from the door.** That setup forces you to pass many other tempting items.

- **Look up and down.** The more expensive items are generally placed at eye level. Bargains can often be found on less-convenient shelves.

- **Become a label reader and use the nutrition information.** A label shows the size of a serving (it may be smaller than you think), the number of servings in the package, and the ingredients, as well as the food's nutrient profile. (See the following section for more information.)

Label Reading 101 for Dieters

Since 1990, when the Food and Drug Administration's Nutrition Labeling and Education Act went into effect, all packaged food products (with a few exceptions) carry labeling, which states the nutrition content in the package. The law also allows manufacturers to use certain food-and-health claims on the labels of their products, too.

But such labeling can be overwhelming. When you understand how to read and use the information on a food label, you'll discover that the label can help you choose foods that fit into your diet. This section explains everything you'll see on a typical label and how to use the information to your advantage.

Nutrition Facts label

Choosing foods wisely based on the information that you can glean from Nutrition Facts labels is key to successful dieting. At first, the label may seem awfully confusing, but if you know what to look for, interpreting a label is really pretty simple.

See the list that follows for the skinny on the most important information featured on the Nutrition Facts label:

- ✔ **Calories:** The calorie total is based on the stated serving size — so if you eat more or less than what the label lists as one portion, you need to do the math.

- ✔ **Dietary fiber:** Choose the foods with the most fiber. Research shows that people who eat plenty of fiber also eat fewer calories. You get the most fiber in foods made from whole grains, such as cereals and breads. Fruits and vegetables have fiber, too. A food is considered to be high in fiber if it has at least 5 grams of fiber per serving.

✔ **Serving size:** Notice how the food manufacturer's serving size compares to the size you usually eat. For example, does your normal serving of ice cream measure more than the standard ½ cup? And remember that serving amounts are given in *level* measuring cups or spoons. Servings per container can help you estimate sizes if a measuring cup or spoon isn't handy.

✔ **Total fat:** For dieting, keep total fat to less than about 20 to 30 percent of calories. For someone who eats 1,500 calories a day, that's no more than 33 to 50 grams. Remember, the Percentage Daily Value numbers on Nutrition Facts labels are based on 65 grams of fat a day (30 percent of total calories) and calculated on a 2,000-calorie-per-day diet.

Trans fatty acid is the newest item to be added to the Nutrition Fact label. Starting in January 2006, all foods required to carry nutrition labeling have to state the amount of trans fatty acids in their product. Like saturated fat, trans fat is a type of fat. The grams of these fats, and their calories, are already accounted for in the total fat.

To quickly figure the number of grams of fat that 30 percent represents, start with your total number of daily calories. Drop the last digit and then divide the remaining number by 3. So if you allow yourself 1,800 calories for the day, divide 180 by 3 to get 60 grams of fat as your daily limit.

More labeling lingo

In addition to the information on the nutrition panel, food packagers can also use descriptive terms, which are very specific and legally defined. Table 5-1 lists some of the terms that are particularly important when on a weight-loss plan.

Table 5-1	Label Lingo
What the Food Label Says	**What It Means**
Fat-free	Less than 0.5 gram of fat in a serving.
Calorie-free	Less than 5 calories per serving.
Low-fat	3 grams of fat (or less) per serving.
Lean (on meat labels)	Less than 10 grams of fat per serving, with 4.5 grams or less of saturated fat and 95 milligrams of cholesterol per serving.
Extra lean (on meat labels)	Less than 5 grams of fat per serving, with less than 2 grams of saturated fat and 95 milligrams of cholesterol.
Less	Contains 25 percent less of a nutrient or calories than another food.
Reduced	A nutritionally altered product that contains at least 25 percent fewer calories, sodium, or sugar than the regular one.
Lite (Light)	Contains one-third fewer calories or no more than half the fat of the higher-calorie, higher-fat version; or no more than half the sodium of the higher-sodium version.
Cholesterol-free	Less than 2 milligrams of cholesterol and 2 grams (or less) of saturated fat per serving.
Healthy	The food must be low in fat and saturated fat and contain limited amounts of cholesterol and sodium.

(continued)

Table 5-1 (continued)

What the Food Label Says	What It Means
Percent fat free	The food must be low in fat or fat free. Plus, it must reflect the amount of fat present in a serving. In other words, if a food contains 5 grams of fat in a serving, it can be labeled "95 percent fat free."
Low-calorie	Fewer than 40 calories per serving

Don't confuse total fat and calories with cholesterol, saturated fat, and sodium. All the nutrients that a food contains are important; however, to achieve weight loss, the total fat and calories are the most important to track. Cholesterol and sodium (salt) don't add calories but eating too much sodium can contribute to water retention and therefore water weight. The calories from saturated fat are included in the *calories from fat* total.

Sneaky Servings and Other Portion Tricks

Many dieters find that portion control is real tricky. Manufacturers certainly don't help in this regard. Some containers look as though they should contain one serving, because that's probably how most people consume them. However, consider that

- ✔ A 16-ounce container of iced tea is 2 servings.

- ✔ A 6½- to 7-ounce can of tuna is 2½ servings.

- ✔ A 4-, 6-, or 8-ounce container of yogurt is considered one serving.

- ✔ A 20-ounce bottle of soda is 2 servings.

See Chapter 4 for tips on estimating portion sizes with your hand.

Chapter 6

Eating Healthfully While Eating Out

. . . .

In This Chapter

▶ Understanding how dining out can add calories

▶ Spotting the high-fat cues on menus

▶ Knowing your best ethnic food choices

. . . .

*E*ating out can pose special problems for dieters. New menu choices are tempting, portion sizes are large, and many professional kitchens don't normally use low-fat or low-calorie cooking methods as standard practice. In fact, as a rule, the less expensive the restaurant, the more likely it is that the kitchen uses generous amounts of fat and high-fat cooking techniques — inexpensive and easy ways to add flavor to food. A fish fillet, for example, must be high quality and cooked skillfully if it's going to taste delicious simply broiled or baked without a coating of oil or buttery sauce.

But don't fear. This chapter can help you navigate menus and still enjoy going out to eat. Armed with the information we give, you can be a dining detective, avoiding the high-fat items and zeroing in on the lower-calorie and lower-fat meals with ease.

Knowing Your Enemy

The whole dining-out experience can cost you plenty
of calories. How many times have you had to wait in
the bar until your table was ready? Cocktails add calories and lessen your diet resolve — you get to the
table famished and not exactly steeled against temptation. And then the impulse to clean your plate over-
takes you because, after all, you're paying big bucks
for the meal. But take heart: You can maneuver
around these predicaments.

For example, if you do dine out frequently, consider becoming a regular at one spot. That way,
the wait staff and kitchen can get to know you.
They can alert you to items that are especially
dieter friendly, and the kitchen won't be thrown
by your special requests — a plus during the
busiest dining hours.

Whether dining out is more special or a routine
part of your day, keep this advice in mind:

- **Restaurant meals are often considered special
  occasions.** More frequently, though, they're last-
  minute solutions when you're too tired or too
  stressed to make dinner. Both scenarios set you
  up for overindulging. Remember to look at the
  meal in context of the entire day's eating or what
  you'll eat over several days.

- **Restaurant meals are often loaded with fat.** Fat
  is an easy way to make foods taste good. Fat is
  also cheap compared to lean meat, so restaurants use it liberally because it makes their
  bottom line healthy — although it doesn't do
  much for the shape of *your* bottom. Be a fat
  detective. Ask questions about preparation and
  request substitutions.

✔ **Portions may be huge.** You often get twice the amount that you really need to eat. Share an entree with a friend or order two appetizers instead of one entree. Don't be embarrassed to ask for a doggie bag.

✔ **Menus are organized with the focus on protein, and the servings of protein are much too large.** Meat, chicken, and fish often get the most "ink," with little attention paid to side dishes. So cast your eye over to the side-dish section and choose from the plainer ones (that is, those without sauces). Another way to create a better balance may be to order your entree from the appetizer section.

✔ **Most meals eaten out include alcohol.** Not only is alcohol calorie heavy and nutrient poor, but it also lowers your resolve to eat healthfully. If you enjoy a cocktail or a glass of wine when eating out, plan to limit your intake to one, and drink it with, not before, the meal.

These are important tactics to keep in mind wherever you dine. They're a start. But menus are always going to be written to entice and seduce you into ordering more than you intend. If you can discover how to read between the lines and spot the red flags for dieters, you'll rarely be duped into ordering and eating more than you want. And when you eat ethnic, try to find out a little about the cuisine, the ingredients, and the typical methods of cooking so that foreign phrases don't throw you.

Menu Sleuthing

If you know how to translate the code, menu descriptions can yield clues to the fat and calorie contents of a dish. For example, "Grande taco salad served in a crispy tortilla shell, topped with lean sautéed ground beef" may sound like a good choice at first. But the words *grande, crispy,* and *sautéed* tell you that this is no low-cal salad. In fact, it contains about 700 calories! If you're restricting your intake to 1,200 calories a day, do you really want to get more than half your calories from a single dish?

Following are the most commonly used menu words that speak volumes — calorically, that is.

Lots of fat:

- ✔ Alfredo
- ✔ Basted
- ✔ Bathed
- ✔ Batter-dipped
- ✔ Breaded
- ✔ Buttery
- ✔ Coated
- ✔ Creamy
- ✔ Crispy and crunchy (except when describing raw vegetables)
- ✔ Deep-fried
- ✔ Dipped
- ✔ Dressed
- ✔ Marinated
- ✔ Pan-fried
- ✔ Rich
- ✔ Sautéed

Huge portion sizes:

- ✔ Combo
- ✔ Feast

(FYI)

A portion to a restaurant may not be a portion to you!

Restaurant portion sizes have more to do with controlling operational expenses than with balancing nutrients. Most restaurants use standardized ladles, spoons, cups, and scoops, and their capacity is generally larger than what you would use at home. Some typical institutional measures are

- ✔ Salad dressing ladle = ¼ cup

- ✔ Pat of butter = 2 teaspoons

- ✔ Scoop of ice cream = 1½ to 2 cups

- ✔ Burger = 6 to 8 ounces

- ✔ Meat, poultry, or fish = 8 to 12 ounces

- ✔ Beverages: small = 2 cups, medium = 4 cups, large = 6 cups

- ✔ Theater popcorn: small = 4 cups, large = 10 cups, jumbo = 15 to 20 cups

- ✔ Wine = 6 to 8 ounces

- ✔ Grande
- ✔ Jumbo
- ✔ King-size
- ✔ Supreme

Saner sizes:

- ✔ Appetizer
- ✔ Kiddie
- ✔ Luncheon

✔ Petite

✔ Regular

✔ Salad-size

Taking a Dieter's Tour of Restaurants

You may think that you must avoid certain types of restaurants or cuisines while you're dieting. Not true. Keep reading if you want to be guided through various cuisines and food scenarios and find out what's "safe" and what's not.

Chinese

Depending on your order, you can get a healthy low-cal meal or a calorie nightmare in a Chinese restaurant; foods are either lean or fatty. Generally, the protein foods in Chinese cuisine — duck, spareribs, and pork — are extremely fatty, although you can also find chicken, shrimp, and lean beef.

Much of the food is deep-fried — even items that may surprise you, such as vegetables in a simple stir-fry are sometimes blanched in hot oil instead of water. And the amount of oil in stir-fries can be staggeringly large.

Family-style dining (large dishes are placed on the table for guests to help themselves) offers another temptation to eat too much simply because the food is there. So start with small portions and have seconds only if you're *really* hungry.

Dieter's aid: Eat the way the Chinese do. Rice is the centerpiece of the meal, and diners eat from their small rice bowls, not from big dinner plates.

Meat and vegetables are selected from the serving dishes, almost one bite at a time, added to the bowl, and eaten with rice. Also, if you can't pass up an especially fatty dish, be sure to balance it with lean ones. Ask for brown rice, which has more fill-you-up fiber.

Choose more of these:

- ✔ Bean curd (unless fried)
- ✔ Fish, shrimp, and scallops
- ✔ Hot and spicy, as opposed to deep-fried
- ✔ Served on a sizzling platter (which means the entrée is broiled or roasted)
- ✔ Vegetables
- ✔ Velvet sauce

Eat less of these:

- ✔ Anything served in a bird's nest
- ✔ Batter-fried foods
- ✔ Breaded and fried foods
- ✔ Crispy noodles on the table
- ✔ Sweet-and-sour dishes
- ✔ Sweet duck sauce
- ✔ Twice-cooked dishes

Delis and sandwich shops

True delicatessens are overly generous on servings, piling sandwiches so high with meat that you need a knife and fork to eat them. What delis do vertically, sub shops (those that sell grinders and hoagies) do horizontally. Therefore, portion control is a must. Menus are usually flexible, so this is one type of restaurant where you can exercise your calorie-smart creativity.

 Dieter's aid: Go to lunch with a friend, split a sandwich, and order an extra roll or bread to make two sandwiches out of the meat in one. Or if you're by yourself, order half a sandwich and extra bread and create two sandwiches for the price of one — taking one home for later, of course. Most restaurants that serve sandwiches also have soup. Order a bowl of a soup made without cream and eat it with an unbuttered roll, and you have a lower-calorie meal.

Choose more of these:

- ✔ Baked or boiled ham
- ✔ Beet salad
- ✔ Carrot and raisin salad
- ✔ Extra tomato, lettuce, and veggies for sandwiches
- ✔ Mustard (not mayo)
- ✔ Pickles
- ✔ Roast or smoked turkey
- ✔ Sauerkraut
- ✔ Sliced chicken (not chicken salad with lots of mayo)
- ✔ Tuna
- ✔ Whole-grain bread

Eat less of these:

- ✔ Bagels (they're huge!)
- ✔ Bologna
- ✔ Corned beef

✔ Eggplant or chicken Parmigiana

✔ Extra cheese

✔ Hot pastrami

✔ Knockwurst

✔ Liverwurst

✔ Meatballs

✔ Mortadella

✔ Reuben sandwiches (grilled corned beef, sauer-kraut, and Swiss cheese with Thousand Island dressing)

✔ Salami

✔ Sausage and peppers

✔ Tongue

Fast food

You can swear never to eat another burger, fry, or shake again, but get real. Often, the one and only option on America's interstates is fast food. And certainly, a trip to the mall usually means passing the food court, with its aromas seducing you to stop for just a little something.

Ever noticed where they put the restrooms in shopping malls? Other than the ones located within department stores, the men's and women's rooms are stacked near the food court. It's no accident — mall designers plan it that way.

 Dieter's aid: To balance all the grim news about fast foods, consider the following few happy thoughts:

✔ **You get no surprises.** You know what will be on the menu. With few exceptions, the menus are the same from coast to coast, so you can choose a restaurant that you know offers items that fit into your diet.

✔ **Except for beverages, portions are generally small, especially if you stick to the regular or kids' sizes.**

✔ **Most restaurants post nutrition information or will provide it when asked, so you can make informed choices.**

Even a small soda is a generous portion, so be sure to order a diet one or a seltzer and drink it all before going back for more food — it *will* fill you up.

Choose more of these:

✔ Baked potato

✔ Fat-free or low-fat milk

✔ Fat-free salad dressing

✔ Grilled chicken

✔ Salad with the dressing on the side

✔ Single burger (regular or kid-size)

✔ Small fries

Eat less of these:

✔ Cheese sauce

✔ Chicken nuggets (they often include the skin)

✔ Croissants

✔ Fish sandwich (it's fried)

✔ Fried chicken

✔ Large and jumbo-size fries

✔ Onion rings

✔ Salad dressing (unless it's fat-free)

✔ Sauces and high-fat add-ons such as cheese, chili, and tartar sauce

✔ Specialty burgers

French

Fat is the pitfall when it comes to French cuisine, from the butter on the table to the cream sauces, rich salad dressings, and desserts. Even lean meats and fish have added fat. Unless the restaurant specializes in *nouvelle cuisine* (the updated style of cooking that relies more on fresh ingredients and less on classic butter-enhanced sauces), you'll be hard-pressed to find diet-friendly foods.

Dieter's aid: Start with an appetite-taming green salad (easy on the dressing) or a clear soup.

Choose more of these:

✔ *Au vapour* (steamed)

✔ *En brochette* (skewered and broiled)

✔ *Grillé* (grilled)

Eat less of these:

✔ *A la crème* (in cream sauce)

✔ *A la mode* (with ice cream)

✔ *Au gratin* or *gratinée* (baked with cheese and cream)

✔ *Crème fraîche* (similar to sour cream)

✔ Drawn butter

✔ *En croûte* (in a pastry crust)

✔ Hollandaise

✔ Puff pastry

✔ *Remoulade* (a mayonnaise-based sauce)

✔ Stuffed

Indian

Some styles of Indian cooking are vegetarian, but don't let that lull you into thinking that these foods are low-cal. Plenty of fat is used in Indian cooking — usually clarified butter called *ghee*. Roasting tandoori style (in a clay oven called a *tandoor*) is a good low-fat cooking method, but other dishes are often stewed and fried. Indian breads are many and varied, ranging from *chapatti* to high-fat, deep-fried *poori*. Often, the chef gives the breads a shimmer of butter before serving them.

Dieter's aid: Indian cuisine doesn't focus on meat; rather, it uses carbohydrates, such as basmati rice (an aromatic long-grain variety) and lentils as its foundation. Vegetables are a part of almost every dish, and the sauces are enriched with yogurt, not cream.

Choose more of these:

✔ Chutney

✔ *Dahl* (lentils)

✔ *Masala* (curry)

✔ *Matta* (peas)

✔ *Paneer* (a fresh milk cheese)

✔ *Pullao* or *pilau* (rice)

✔ *Raita* (a yogurt and cucumber condiment)

Eat less of these:

✔ Chickpea batter used to deep-fry

✔ *Ghee* (clarified butter)

✔ *Korma* (cream sauce)

✔ *Molee* (coconut)

✔ *Poori* (a deep-fried bread)

✔ *Samosas* (fried turnover appetizers)

Italian

Most Americans think of heavy southern Italian food when they think of high-cal items: meatballs, eggplant Parmigiana, veal Parmigiana, and lasagna. However, the food of northern Italy, while it may appear less caloric, also has its detractors: butter, olive oil, and cream.

Dieter's aid: Portions are overly generous in most Italian restaurants, so this may be a good place for sharing — particularly important when you consider that an antipasto of cheese, marinated vegetables, salami, and garlic bread can use up a day's calorie budget before the main course arrives. Bread on the table served with butter or olive oil can be a diet buster. Ask for tomato sauce for dipping if you must fill up on bread and have the fats removed. Or better yet, out of sight, out of mouth; have the bread removed, too. Order vegetables à la carte as long as they're not cooked with plenty of fat or deep-fried. And instead of a creamy dessert, order a low-fat cappuccino with fruit.

Choose more of these:

✔ Light red sauce

✔ Marinara sauce

✔ Pasta (other than those stuffed with cheese)

✔ *Piccata* (lemon-wine sauce)

✔ White or red clam sauce (but ask the wait staff; some clam sauces are made with cream)

✔ Wine sauce

Eat less of these:

✔ Alfredo

✔ *Alla panna* (with cream)

✔ Butter

✔ *Carbonara* (butter, eggs, bacon, and sometimes cream sauce)

✔ Fried eggplant or zucchini

✔ *Frito misto* (fried mixed vegetables or seafood)

✔ Olive oil

✔ *Parmigiana* (baked in sauce with cheese)

✔ Prosciutto

✔ Salami

Japanese

Japanese can be one of the healthiest cuisines, with only a few fattening dishes, such as tempura, teriyaki, katso, and sukiyaki. If eaten in the balance that the Japanese apply — heavy on the vegetables and light on the fats and meats — Japanese food can be a dieter's dream.

Dieter's aid: Portions are small, and rice and noodles are the foundation. Cooking techniques are most often broiling, steaming, braising, or simmering — all of which generally produce low-cal and low-fat dishes.

Choose more of these:

✔ Clear broth

✔ *Miso* (fermented soy)

✔ *Miso* dressing

✔ *Mushimono* (steamed)

✔ *Nabemono* (a one-pot dish)

✔ *Nimono* (simmered)

✔ Sashimi

✔ Sushi

✔ *Udon* (noodles)

✔ *Yaki* (broiled)

✔ *Yakimono* (grilled)

Eat less of these:

✔ *Agemono* (deep-fried)

✔ *Katsu* (fried pork cutlet)

✔ *Sukiyaki* (a one-dish meal made with fatty beef)

✔ *Tempura* (batter-fried)

Mexican

The good news is that Mexican cuisine places minimal emphasis on meat protein. The bad news is that most Mexican food is fried or cooked in abundant amounts of fat.

For example, a flour tortilla is fine on its own, but roll it around a filling and deep-fry it, and you have *mucho calorica.* Many of the national Mexican food chains don't use lard or animal fat drippings, which is typical in many independent restaurants, but they do use

plenty of vegetable oil. As far as calories are con-
cerned, there's no difference between animal fat and
vegetable fat.

 Dieter's aid: Use salsa instead of salad dressing,
guacamole, or sour cream on entrees. Ask for
cheese toppings to be omitted or ask if low-fat
sour cream and cheese are available.

Choose more of these:

- Black bean soup
- *Ceviche* (fish or scallops marinated in lime juice)
- Chili
- Enchiladas, burritos, or soft tacos (skip the sour cream, guacamole, and most of the cheese)
- Fajitas
- Gazpacho
- Mexican salad minus the fried taco shell

Eat less of these:

- Chimichangas
- Extra cheese
- Refried beans
- Sour cream
- Tortilla shells

Pizza

The trend toward newfangled pizza is a real plus for
dieters. You can add or subtract ingredients to fit your
particular tastes. Meat choices have moved from extra
pepperoni, sausage, and bacon to grilled chicken and
shrimp. You can specify the kind of cheese you like

and replace high-fat, low-flavor mozzarella with a smaller amount of full-flavored goat cheese or feta. Even a traditional pizzeria can be diet friendly if you order selectively.

 Dieter's aid: If you can, start with a small salad to take the edge off your appetite. Order it with the dressing on the side or extra vinegar to thin it.

Choose more of these:

- ✔ Canadian bacon
- ✔ Grilled chicken
- ✔ Part-skim cheeses, or strongly flavored ones
- ✔ Shrimp
- ✔ Tuna
- ✔ Vegetable toppings, especially broccoli and spinach

Eat less of these:

- ✔ Bacon
- ✔ Extra cheese
- ✔ Extra olive oil
- ✔ Meatballs
- ✔ Olives
- ✔ Pepperoni
- ✔ Sausage

Thai

Light on fats, most Thai dishes are stir-fried, steamed, braised, or marinated. The one exception is Thai curry, which is made with coconut milk. It's loaded with calories — 1 cup of the milk contains 445 calories.

PRO SPEAK

Low calorie by law

You can be sure that you're getting a low-calorie meal when you order one. The Food and Drug Administration (FDA) has ruled that all restaurants (including airlines) must demonstrate that special menus comply with the same federal regulations as those used on the labels of packaged foods.

The only difference is that restaurateurs aren't held to the same grueling standards applied to food manufacturers. They're not required to do laboratory nutrition analysis — they can use computer programs to do their calculations and show that the menu items are prepared from recipes that comply with the standards. They don't have to post the nutrient contents of their food, but they must have it available if you ask.

If you see these terms on a menu, they must comply with FDA standards.

✔ **Low calorie:** It contains 120 calories or less per 100 grams (about 3½ ounces).

✔ **Low-fat:** It has less than 3 grams of fat per 100 grams.

✔ **Low-cholesterol:** These items must contain less than 20 milligrams of cholesterol per 100 grams and no more than 2 grams of saturated fat.

✔ **Low sodium:** It has 140 milligrams or less of sodium per 100 grams.

✔ **Light:** This means that the item is low in fat or calories. (Restaurants may continue to use the term *light* as in "Lighter Fare" to mean smaller portions, as long as they make it clear how they're using the word.)

✔ **Healthy:** It's low in fat and saturated fat, has limited amounts of cholesterol and sodium, and provides significant amounts of one or more key nutrients: vitamin A, vitamin C, iron, calcium, protein, or fiber.

Dieter's aid: Rice and noodles are staples. Ask the chef to substitute leaner scallops, shrimp, or skinless chicken for fatty duck. The ingredients in many Thai dishes are interchangeable, so asking for substitutions shouldn't pose a problem.

Choose more of these:

- ✔ Basil sauce
- ✔ Bean thread noodles
- ✔ Fish sauce
- ✔ Lime sauce
- ✔ *Sâté* (skewered and grilled meats)
- ✔ Sizzling
- ✔ Thai salad

Eat less of these:

- ✔ Coconut milk soup
- ✔ *Mee-krob* (crispy noodles)
- ✔ Peanut sauce
- ✔ Red, green, and yellow mussman curries (they contain coconut milk)

Chapter 7

Joining a Weight-Loss Program

. . . .

In This Chapter

▶ Determining whether you need an organized group

▶ Sorting out the ragtag from the bobtail programs

▶ Going online and deciding what's right for you

. . . .

*I*f you're reading this chapter, chances are you're wondering if the support of an organized group is the kind of commitment that you require. This chapter shows you how these programs compare and gives you the background ammunition that you need to sort through the maze of options.

The programs are grouped in categories based on the kinds of support they offer. Some require more visits than others, some cost an arm and a leg and some are fairly reasonable, and some are more restrictive than others. You can find self-help groups that offer only support, not concrete diet or exercise advice. Others require membership and the purchase of special foods or meal replacements.

The big news in weight-loss support is the growth of online plans. Many programs that may have been geographically off limits in the past can now be accessed through the convenience of your computer — but don't just let your fingers do the walking — move your legs, too! Plus, you can find a crop of new Web-only programs that are worth a look. I give you the lowdown on these in this chapter as well.

Don't think that one of the programs listed in this chapter has all the magic that you're seeking. Two extremely large surveys suggest that weight-loss programs may not hold the key to successful weight loss and maintenance. *Consumer Reports* conducted a 2002 investigation revealing that of the 8,000 people who lost at least 10 percent of their starting weight and kept it off for at least one year (the official definition of weight-loss success), a stunning 83 percent of them lost weight without help. And, half of the members of the National Weight Control Registry — a database maintained by the University of Colorado of about 3,000 successful dieters — did *not* use outside help.

That doesn't mean that you should turn your back on the help available. Although in the minority, some successful losers *did* find the extra support critical to their success.

Finding a Good Fit from the Start

One size never fits all. So before you sign up for a weight-loss program, ask yourself the following questions. You may not be able to answer all of them with certainty, but do keep these points in mind as you weigh your options:

- ✔ Do I need the support of a group to keep me going?

- ✔ Do I have the time to commit to attending weekly sessions or meetings for up to a year?

✔ Can I afford to join a club or program?

✔ Does the program require special foods and can I afford them? If so, will my eating special foods interfere with my family's lifestyle?

✔ Am I willing to follow a program's instructions, guidance, and skill-building techniques to find out how to eat in a more healthful way and, if the program requires it, be physically active for the long term?

Meal-Plan-Based Programs

Weight-loss programs based on meal plans can be good options for people who have trouble sticking to a weight-loss plan on their own. A 2003 report in the *Journal of the American Medical Association* concluded that the structure of commercial programs gave some dieters an advantage that resulted in more weight loss than dieters who attended self-help programs.

Meal-based programs offer a variety of services, from special foods and custom-designed diets and exercise programs to liquids only. Having so many choices can be confusing, however — and sitting in the office of a recruiter for one of these programs can be intimidating. (Recruiters are salespeople, well trained at closing a deal.) By carefully evaluating the programs in this section, you can avoid signing up and then not showing up because you hate the foods that you must eat or because the plan doesn't provide enough supervision.

Jenny Craig, Inc.

Philosophy: The program is based on exercise, lifestyle modification, and a low-calorie diet. Members are advised to eat three meals and three snacks a day and increase physical activity. Prepared packaged foods are available and encouraged especially during the initial phases of weight loss. Rapid weight loss is discouraged. Expected weight loss is 1 to 2 pounds per week.

Staff: Registered dietitians design the programs and trained, nonmedical personnel administer them. The nonmedicals must complete a 56-hour training session and participate in monthly continuing education sessions.

Cost: Programs and specials vary but generally cost $1 per pound. The food is extra. A one-time enroll-ment fee is required. The initial weight-loss plan requires that you use their foods, which costs an additional $75 a week.

Availability: Centers are located in 46 states and in Puerto Rico, Canada, Australia, and New Zealand. The program can be accessed via the Web.

Contact:
11355 North Torrey Rd.
La Jolla, CA 92038-7910
Phone: 800-597-JENNY
Web: www.jennycraig.com

Weight Watchers

Philosophy: Diets are individualized and are based on a point system instead of calorie counting. Point tar-gets are assigned based on your current weight. You can choose any food you want to eat each day as long as you don't go over your targeted number of points. You can "earn" extra points by exercising. Commercial Weight Watchers food products can be purchased but are optional for program participation. Expected weight loss is 1 to 2 pounds per week. Members can stay enrolled for as long as it takes them to reach their goals. Exercise is encouraged, and group counseling sessions are included. Lifestyle modification is a component of the overall program structure.

Staff: Registered dietitians, exercise physiologists, and clinical psychologists developed this program. Leaders (who are Lifetime Members) deliver the program; their initial training requires at least 46 hours of classroom instruction.

Cost: For weight loss, you pay a one-time registration fee of $16 to $20 and a weekly fee of $10 to $14. For maintenance, the fee is $10 to $14 weekly for about six weeks until Lifetime Member status is reached. Lifetime Members don't pay a fee.

Availability: In North America, 20,000 weekly meetings take place. To find a meeting, use the meeting finder feature on the Weight Watchers Web site. Simply type in your zip code for a list of locations near you. Online meetings are also available.

Contact:
175 Crossways Park West
Woodbury, NY 11797
Phone: 800-651-6000
Web: www.weight-watchers.com

Health Management Resources (HMR)

Philosophy: This is a medically supervised rapid weight-loss program for moderate or high-risk weight-loss patients. It's administered in hospitals and health-care settings. Participants who use a very-low-calorie diet (VLCD) of about 500 to 800 calories a day must be under the care of medical personnel. A second option of a 1,200-calorie-a-day diet is also offered. Both plans require meal-replacement shakes, entrees, and bars. Weekly 90-minute classes are mandatory. Expected weight loss is 1 to 5 pounds per week. Medical screening is required for all participants.

Staff: Physicians, registered dietitians, registered nurses, and psychologists developed the program. Programs offering the VLCD have an MD, RN, and health educator on staff.

Comments: The side effects of a very-low-calorie diet may include intolerance to cold, constipation, dizziness, dry skin, and headaches.

 A complication of some of the VLCD programs is gallbladder stones. This is due to the very-low-fat nature of the diets and the fact that the individuals who go on these programs tend to be very overweight and are predisposed to developing stones.

Cost: Fees vary. Healthy Solutions program fees average $20 per week (shakes and entrees are additional). The VLCD averages $50 a week. Maintenance costs average $80 per month.

Availability: The program is available at more than 200 hospitals and medical settings in the United States.

Contact:
59 Temple Place, Suite 704
Boston, MA 02111
Phone: 800-418-1367
Web: www.yourbetterhealth.com

Optifast
Philosophy: This medically supervised rapid weight-loss program is administered in hospitals and clinics. The plan requires liquid meal replacements and/or

fortified food bars. As weight loss progresses, more regular foods are added. Dieters are assigned to an 800-, 950-, or 1,200-calorie plan. Participation is limited to individuals who must lose at least 50 pounds. The weight-loss portion of the program lasts about three months and transition takes six weeks; participants are transitioned to maintenance after five months. Emphasis is on behavior modification, problem-solving skills, physical activity, and individual counseling.

Staff: Group meeting leaders and one-on-one counselors are psychologists or dietitians. Physicians, registered nurses, registered dietitians, and psychologists regularly see each dieter at most locations.

Comments: Be aware that long-term weight-loss maintenance on VLCDs is disappointing. Although participants initially achieve impressive losses, after five years, the majority of patients regain all their weight.

Cost: Costs range from $1,500 to $3,000 for the six-month program. The price may include maintenance at some centers.

Availability: The program is available in numerous hospitals and clinics in the United States and Canada. Residents in the United States can find a clinic on the Optifast Web site by typing in their area codes and zip codes. Residents of Canada can call 800-986-3855, ext. 4067, for clinic locations.

Contact:
Novartis Nutrition
1441 Park Place Blvd.
Minneapolis, MN 55416
Phone: 800-662-2540
Web: www.optifast.com

Non-Diet Programs and Support Groups

Often, the real problems that dieters face aren't only what they eat but *why* they eat the way that they do. The following programs focus on the nonfood factors that may contribute to obesity and stand in the way of weight-loss success. If you could use some peer support while trying to lose weight — but don't require a regimented plan structure or the services of program-provided weight-loss professionals — one of the organizations in this section may be your best choice.

The Solution

Philosophy: The focus of the program is on developing internal skills of self-nurturing and setting limits to achieve balance and freedom from excess. There is a diet plan based on government recommendations and recommendations for exercise. Laurel Mellin, MA, RD, developed the program from her books, *The Solution* and *The Pathway*. The program has been refined to include community and professional support.

Staff: Most providers are mental-health professionals or registered dietitians; all are "Solution Certified," meaning that they have completed and passed special training classes. The program delivery team consists of registered dietitians and licensed mental-health professionals (psychologists, family therapists, social workers, and psychiatrists).

Comments: During the maintenance program, clients can return for 12-week sessions at any time. Every three months, a Saturday afternoon maintenance session for all program graduates is held.

Cost: Materials must be ordered from the center and costs start at about $100. The initial fees for support groups (four weekly, two-hour sessions) are about $150. Cost can run from $250 to $600, depending on needs. The books on which the program is based can be purchased at bookstores.

Availability: Coursework is done in group meetings and coaching sessions, though the workbooks can be purchased and used privately. One hundred fifty groups meet all over the United States. The program also offers telegroups and telecoaching through video-conferencing centers.

Contact:
The Institute for Health Solutions
1623A Fifth Ave.
San Rafael, CA 94901
Phone: 415-457-3331
Web: www.sweetestfruit.org

Overeaters Anonymous (OA)

Philosophy: Overeaters Anonymous is based on the 12 steps of Alcoholics Anonymous, a proven model that has helped millions of people with addictive behaviors. The group recommends emotional, spiritual, and physical recovery changes. It makes no exercise or food recommendations.

Staff: Volunteer group leaders who meet specific criteria run the meetings. No healthcare providers are on staff.

Cost: You have no dues or fees. The group is self-supporting through member contributions.

Availability: Groups meet in more than 50 countries in churches, hospitals, and rehab centers.

Contact:
World Service Office (WSO)
6075 Zenith Court NE
Rio Rancho, NM 87124
Phone: 505-891-2664
Web: www.oa.org

TOPS Club, Inc. (Taking Off Pounds Sensibly)

Philosophy: The desire to change comes from within; a supporting environment provides the most effective way to sustain change. The group doesn't impose or set weight-loss goals other than the ones you bring to the group. The group encourages you to remain a part of TOPS as long as you need support.

Staff: Each chapter is lead by a volunteer leader. A nine-member board of directors administers the program, and a field staff of regional directors, coordinators, and area captains supports the volunteer chapter leaders.

Cost: Annual membership is $20 in the United States and $25 in Canada. This amount includes the monthly magazine. Local chapters charge nominal fees of 50¢ to $1 per week.

Availability: Two hundred and thirty thousand members meet weekly in 10,300 chapters in the United States, Canada, and around the world. Online membership is available.

Contact:
4575 S. Fifth St.
Milwaukee, WI 53207
Phone: 800-932-8677
Web: www.tops.org

Overcoming Overeating (OO)

Philosophy: Compulsive eaters are people preoccupied with food to the extent that it has become self-destructive. They believe that dieting has not solved weight problems but caused compulsive overeating. Change comes from self-acceptance and weight acceptance. They don't address eating disorders.

Staff: Codirectors Jane R. Hirschmann, MSW, a psychotherapist, and Carol H. Munter, a psychoanalyst, are specialists in eating disorders. The program is based on their 1998 book, *Overcoming Overeating*. Trained social workers or psychologists run programs located outside of New York City.

Cost: Workshops run about $45. Private-session fees are based on a sliding scale; group-meeting fees are $25 to $45 and are set by the individual therapist. Audio and videotapes can be ordered for $39.95 and $119.95 respectively, plus shipping and handling.

Availability: Centers are located in New York, Chicago, and New England. A referral list by therapist's state and support groups is posted on their Web site. Online e-mail chat groups are ongoing and online chat relays are frequently scheduled.

Contact:
National Center for Overcoming Overeating
P.O. Box 1257
Old Chelsea Station
New York, NY 10113-0920
Phone: 212-875-0442
Web: www.overcomingovereating.com

Online and E-Mail Programs

The biggest news for diet help is online access to programs. Could they be an aid to your success?

Researchers wondered that, too. And as two studies (one in 2001 and one in April 2003) in the *Journal of the American Medical Association* report, the answer is a definite yes, especially if the plans incorporate e-mail with behavioral advice and support.

Keep in mind, plenty of junk science is out there, but the sites that follow are the best.

Nutrio.com

Philosophy: A site that offers expert weight-loss and weight-management assessments, tools, and resources with private and community message boards.

Staff: A team of registered dietitians, exercise physiologists, and therapists designed and maintain the site.

Cost: Free content is general. Subscription service ($10 activation plus $9.95 a month; discounts available for annual membership) offers one-on-one counseling on nutrition and fitness. Recipes, shopping lists, dining-out guides, and customized meal plans are available. Subscribers can log their nutrition and fitness progress.

Contact:
Nutrio.com
2843 Executive Park Dr.
Weston, FL 33331
Phone: 954-385-4700
Web: www.nutrio.com

DietingPlans.com

Philosophy: An interactive site that offers expert diet planning, fitness, and one-on-one support from dietitians. Thirty minutes of aerobic activity on three or more days a week is expected. The diet plan is based on the member's personal diet profile, and a virtual trainer aids physical activity.

Staff: Dietitians staff the site for one-on-one sessions, and they also answer e-mail.

Cost: Subscription is $14.95 per month.

Contact:
6060 Center Dr.
Los Angeles, CA 90045
Phone: 800-269-4390
Web: www.dietingplans.com

NutriTeen.com

Philosophy: A site geared to 12- to 17-year olds. Each person is given a personal counselor, a dietitian, and a personal trainer who e-mails support and coaching. Parents are required to participate in a separate, integrated program. The plan includes behavior modification, eating healthfully as opposed to a weight-loss diet, and physical activity. The program lasts 12 months.

Staff: A board of pediatric doctors, psychologists, dietitians, and fitness experts supervises the program. Registered Dietitians and Certified Personal Fitness Trainers counsel the children.

Cost: $99 for a three-month membership.

Contact:
NutriTeen
P.O. Box 1272
Old Chelsea Station
New York, NY 10113
Phone: 866-LOSE-123
Web: www.nutriteen.com

Cyberdiet.net

Philosophy: Members receive meal plans and can follow their eating and exercise progress. The site has plenty of information on diet, nutrition, and fitness. Members can access a community of fellow dieters through an online message board and online chats.

Staff: The director of nutrition services is a registered dietitian.

Cost: The initial charge of $39.95 covers membership (the fee includes a $10 registration fee) for two months. Then, thereafter, the monthly fee is $14.95.

Contact:
DietWatch.com, Inc.
336 Atlantic Ave, Suite 301
East Rockaway, NY 11518
Web: www.cyberdiet.net

Determining Which Program Is Right for You

After you consider the different types of weight-loss programs and find one that you think may work for you, make an appointment to visit one of that program's centers for a personal interview. Take along the following list of questions and demand satisfying answers. (You may already know some of the answers based on the information given in this chapter, but having the program reconfirm that information certainly doesn't hurt.) How truthfully and in how straightforward a manner the answers are given can help you decide whether a particular program is right for you.

✔ What data proves that the program actually works? What has been written about the program's success, besides individual testimonials?

✔ Do customers keep off the weight after they leave the diet program? (Ask for results over two to five years. The Federal Trade Commission requires weight-loss companies to back up their claims.)

✔ What are the program's requirements? Are special menus or foods, counseling visits, or exercise a part of the program?

✔ Does the plan include physical activity recommendations? Will the program include guidance on physical activity for the long term? How?

✔ What are the approaches and goals of the program?

✔ What are the health risks?

✔ If I don't need to purchase special meals, does the plan take into account my personal food preferences? Will I have to give up all my favorite foods? Are the foods available at the supermarket? Will the program help me to discover how to live with its eating plan for the long term? How?

✔ What are the costs of membership, weekly fees, food, supplements, maintenance, and counseling? What's the payment schedule? Are any costs covered under health insurance? Will the organization give a refund if I drop out or give rebates for successful weight loss and maintenance?

✔ Will the staff monitor my success at three- to six-month intervals and then modify the program if needed?

✔ Does the plan have a maintenance program? Is it part of the package or does it cost extra?

✔ What kind of professional support is provided? What are the credentials and experiences of these professionals? (Detailed information should be available on request.)

Chapter 8

Ten Strategies to Keep the Weight Off

*W*e hope that you've made some good progress with your weight-loss program and that you're eager not to lose ground. A weight-maintenance program should be a priority after the initial six months of a weight-loss diet. Weight maintenance isn't a matter of "going off your diet" — it's a matter of keeping your eating and activity habits up to a healthy standard.

In some ways, the strategies you need for maintenance are no different from those that you used to lose weight in the first place. But in other ways, the strategies *are* different. Maintenance means keeping at it forever. Stop, and you'll slide right back up to where you started — or worse yet, even higher.

To maintain a healthy weight, you must maintain a healthy lifestyle — balancing your diet with exercise, stress reduction, and relationships in a healthy manner. As you work through your weight-loss plan and look forward to staying at your new, lower weight, consider the points in this chapter. They're the real measures of a healthy weight.

Be Realistic

Assigning a number as your ideal weight, based on information from a height-and-weight chart, isn't really a healthy way to judge your progress. Although the charts do serve a useful purpose as guides to a healthy weight range, specifying a number as *ideal* connotes that any number higher than that isn't good enough. Establishing an ideal weight sets you up in pass/fail mode instead of giving you credit for

Have you reached a reasonable weight for you?

If you have your heart set on a particular point on the scale that's lower than you are now, ask yourself how reasonable it is for you to reach and maintain that weight. You can answer that question by looking at your current weight-loss success and your diet history. Ask yourself the following questions:

✔ What's the lowest adult weight you were able to maintain for at least one year?

✔ Think of a time that you were at a lower weight than you are now. How difficult was it to reach that weight and stay there? How much exercise did you have to do? How few calories did you have to eat?

✔ Considering your starting weight and clothing size, what's the largest clothing size in which you feel comfortable and think that you look pretty good?

progress made. Thinking of your weight in terms of what's *reasonable* for you is healthier.

For more information about adjusting your attitude and getting realistic about your weight, see Chapter 2.

Be Adventurous

Changing your attitude about yourself and your body may be the most beneficial step you can take. If your weight keeps you from enjoying activities, let the issue go.

Have you ever said, "I'll go on vacation when I'm 125 pounds again" or "I'll try water-skiing when I'm thinner" or "I'll go for a hike in the woods when I'm in better shape"? Don't wait until you reach your goal weight. If you do, you're missing out on plenty of living.

Don't miss out on life, because you're hiding behind your weight. You can try many activities no matter what your weight — inline skating, ballroom dancing, ice skating, skiing, hiking, or biking, just to name a few.

 Be adventurous with your eating as well as with your activities. Try a new fruit that you've never tasted. If you always eat bananas and apples but are so bored with them that you don't eat your recommended number of fruit servings, break out of your rut. Try a papaya or a kiwi. Reach for different grains, too. White, long-grain rice is nice, but don't miss out on the short, medium, aromatic, and brown rice varieties. And then you have *quinoa* (pronounced *keen*-wa), barley, and cracked wheat. Experiment with recipes.

Be Flexible

You need to be flexible about what you consider to be weight-loss success. You also need to be flexible about what you consider to be a successful dieting or exercise day. Sure, you need to set goals, but you also need to accept that some days you aren't going to make them. Adding a week's worth of healthy meals and exercise to another week and another and another — even if you don't meet your goal on a few days in between — is how you build success.

 If you can't work in your normal walking route one day, try to stay active in other ways. For example, park your car in the parking space that's farthest from the door. Be sure to take the stairs rather than the elevator. Any kind of exercise counts. If you're stuck at a family party or business meal and every dish in sight is a caloric disaster, don't throw in the towel and overeat. Enjoy small amounts of the foods that are offered and then be especially diligent at the next meal or the next day.

Be Sensible

"I'm never going to eat another pepperoni pizza again!" Doesn't that sound silly? Ban words like *never* and *always* from your eating and exercise plans. These ultimatums put you just bites away from failure. Better to have one small serving and enjoy every bit or share a serving with a friend or pack half of it in a doggie bag for another meal on another day.

Exercising a little every day is better than trying to make up for a missed day or week by overexerting yourself. Chances are, you won't enjoy the exercise as much if you're overdoing it, and you'll probably be so sore afterward that you'll miss the next few days of activity as well. No pain, no gain isn't our motto. Take it slow and steady and *enjoy* yourself — that's what's most important.

Be Active

Don't you just love folks who say things like "We won the baseball game," when they mean that the team they were rooting for on TV won? Or the people who say that they're going to walk the dog and then go outside and watch the dog walk around the yard while they stand in the driveway? These people are spectators, not participants.

We use many other expressions that make us sound active: "Mow the lawn" (or do we sit on the mower?); "wash the clothes" (or do we put them into the washing machine?); "shovel the snow" (or do we push the snow blower?); "run to the store" (or do we drive the car?) — you get the idea. These passive activities sound like actions, but they're really not.

 If you're guilty of using more active language than actually being active, change your behavior. Look for ways — big and small — to fit activity into your day: Climb the stairs, hide the remote, don't use your kids as slaves to fetch things, walk during your lunch break instead of sitting, play ball instead of watching, walk to the school bus stop instead of driving to meet the kids. Park farther from the store instead of circling to find the closest spot, and toss the remote.

Try, Try, and Try Again

The average woman goes on 15 diets in her lifetime and loses about 100 pounds. But she regains
about 125! Experts call it *yo-yo dieting* or *weight
cycling*. At one time, health authorities believed
that each time a person's weight yo-yos, weight
loss becomes more difficult in the future. The

Is yo-yo dieting a no-no?

Yo-yo dieting is going on and off and on and off a diet so that
weight goes up and down the scale, bouncing from one
weight to another. After finding that rats who lost and
regained weight had more body fat than those whose
weights remained stable, researchers concluded that the
more humans diet to lose weight, the less healthy they
become. But a subsequent review of that study and many
other studies proved otherwise. The entire body of research
concludes that yo-yo dieting does *not*

✔ Make future weight loss more difficult.

✔ Increase body fat.

✔ Change the location where body fat is stored.

✔ Lower energy expenditure.

✔ Increase preference for fatty foods.

✔ Change blood pressure.

✔ Change blood cholesterol or triglycerides.

✔ Change insulin or glucose metabolism.

However, the psychological effects of weight cycling can
be distressing. Some research has found that weight
cyclers who tend to binge, binge more when they cycle.

individual loses more muscle, needs fewer calories to maintain the weight, and becomes more frustrated. The bottom line seemed to be that you're better off not trying to lose weight and that going on repeated diets is dangerous.

One major study published in the *Journal of the American Medical Association* looked at 43 studies and found no convincing evidence that weight cycling in humans has adverse health effects on body composition, energy balance, risk factors for cardiovascular disease, or the success of future efforts at weight loss. Proof positive is the fact that 90 percent of the people in the National Weight Control Registry had tried to lose weight previously — in fact, each person had lost and regained an average of 270 pounds! Yet they were able to lose weight and keep it off, once and for all — even after years of yo-yo dieting.

Weigh In

When you're trying to maintain weight loss, monitoring your weight closely is the best approach. Successful maintainers are able to catch a 5- or 10-pound weight creep and take immediate action. Many people in the National Weight Control Registry say that they weigh themselves every day. During the weight-loss phase, weighing daily can be disappointing, so experts recommend that you get on the scale no more than once a week. But when you're in maintenance, you may find it helpful to more closely monitor the scale so that you can make adjustments to your eating plan before a 1- or 2-pound gain becomes the 5 pounds you just can't seem to lose.

 During your maintenance phase, continue to weigh in, so to speak, on what you eat, too. Some successful maintainers continue to monitor what they eat by keeping food records. And they stick with a low-fat, low-calorie eating plan.

Solve Problems

People who can keep their weight stable are good problem solvers. They find ways to fit exercise into their schedules. They uncover techniques to eat low-fat foods. They work balance and moderation into their eating plans and exercise routines.

Move

Physical activity is a key predictor of weight-loss maintenance success. Besides helping you to lose weight, regular physical activity is a super stress reducer. (Less stress means less eating in response to stress.) You'll have more energy, not less. (Many people eat when they're dragging and feeling tired.) If you walk with a friend, you'll have good quality time, too.

Don't try to make up for a slow day with an overly active one. But if you do go overboard with an activity that's too strenuous, still try to do something the next day, even if it means a slow walk. The important thing is to do some kind of exercise every day. That's how you make it a habit.

Get Support

You can't lose weight without support nor can you maintain your loss without help. Most successful weight losers are motivated by their own personal needs, but they do have support from friends, spouses, family, or a group of like-minded dieters. They can turn to these people for help with managing the stress in their lives, solving problems, and scheduling time for exercise by handing off household or child-care responsibilities. People who lend support also can serve as cheerleaders and provide attaboy (or attagirl) encouragement. Don't go it alone!

Be a team player

People are social animals. After all, what's the purpose of life if not to be in relationships with other people? Finding someone to lean on is important. But in order to get support, you must give it as well. Maybe your support person is not a fellow dieter, but he needs to rely on you sometimes, too. You can't take without giving, or your support will walk.

Follow these tips to be a good team player:

✔ **Show up.** Whether you make plans to meet your support person at a regular time or you have a more relaxed and informal arrangement, be there. Don't have other activities planned that take away from the agenda. You're there for each other, so be there in mind, body, and spirit.

✔ **Really listen.** Listening takes effort. A phone call can work sometimes. But if possible, meet the other person and talk face to face. See the person as well as hear his words. Visual clues can yield plenty of information. Look for expressions or body language that supports or contradicts what you're hearing.

✔ **Don't judge.** Maybe what you're hearing sounds silly or just plain dumb. But hang in there. When your partner tells you that there's no time to exercise, the judgmental response is, "You're looking for excuses." The nonjudgmental reaction is, "What would make it easier for you to find the time?" Nonjudgmental statements are supportive and lead to discussion. Judgmental ones are conversation stoppers.

✔ **Be supportive.** Offer moral support by showing that you understand. Share similar experiences and give constructive suggestions if you can think of ways to help.

Ten Best Ways to Train Your Core

• •

In This Chapter

▶ Getting on the ball

▶ Moving for core strength

▶ Stretching your muscles

• •

A weak back is your body's way of telling you that your abs are weak. Your back and abs go hand in hand — together they make up your core. Think of core training as preventive medicine that creates balance between your back and abs, and returns your body to its natural, pain-free state.

This bonus excerpt from *Core Strength For Dummies* gives you ten fast and fun ways to shore up your core. You can do the exercises outdoors or with a partner to make them more interesting and fun. And if you want more great tips, check out *Core Strength For Dummies,* available at a bookstore near you or by going to www.dummies.com!

Balance It

Here's an amazing exercise you can do with your exercise ball without even trying; you won't even break a sweat! Sit on your exercise ball instead of in your office chair for just one hour a day and you'll get tighter abs and a stronger back! Just by sitting up straight and sucking in your tummy, you improve your core strength and your balance at the same time. To keep from falling off the ball, you have to keep your feet flat on the floor and pull your abs in tight. Because the ball is round, you can't just plop yourself into it any old way like you can in a chair. See where I'm going with this? You're forced to strengthen your core.

Crunch It

One of the most effective methods for relieving belly fat and strengthening those abs is crunching them! Bringing your upper body to your lower body trains both the upper and lower parts of your abdominal muscles.

Here's an easy yet effective crunch: Grab an exercise ball and lie on the floor with your knees bent and feet flat on the floor and your arms behind your head. Place the ball between your ankles and bring your upper body to your lower body, or bring your knees toward your elbows. This crunch works both your upper and lower abs and is much easier to do than a conventional ball sit-up.

Fix It with Cardio

The best prevention against tummy fat is to stay low in body fat — and that means less belly fat. Doing 60 minutes of cardio exercise at least three times a week helps you maintain a low percentage of body fat, which in turn helps your six-pack peek through.

Jumping rope for 5 to 10 minutes at a time does the trick (ever see a boxer with belly fat?) and also helps keep your joints flexible. Or you can use a mini-trampoline like the Reebok Rebounder to do cardio that also helps train your abs and back. As you perform small bounces on the trampoline, your circulation increases to help flush out fatty deposits in your legs and your belly area.

Other great forms of cardio are running sprints, doing jumping jacks, or performing other activities that get your heart rate elevated and can be done consistently for at least 30 minutes. In fact, try to work in 30 minutes of cardio a day, five days a week if a full 60 minutes, three days a week just doesn't leave you enough time; you'll get the same results. Remember, consistency is the key!

Stretch It Out

Whether you lead a sedentary lifestyle or are an elite athlete, tight muscles in your abs, hips, back, and buttocks can put so much strain and stress on your lower back that the end result is low back pain. One solution that has been proven to be effective is regular stretching. Check out the bonus chapter following this one for some great stretches that are easy to incorporate into your everyday life. Never forget — a healthy core is a strong and flexible back.

Walk It Out

If you want to banish belly fat and strengthen your core, but rigorous exercise is the last activity you want to add to your routine, take a walk every night after dinner.

Walking is the best form of exercise for getting rid of belly fat and training your core (and you'll enjoy your neighborhood at the same time). When you take long strides, you work all the muscles that support your stomach, back, and pelvis. Plus walking is easy to do, and you only need to do it 30 minutes a day, five days a week. Trust me, it works better than skipping dessert (although that doesn't hurt!).

Cycle through It

When you're cycling, you use your legs to spin the wheel and your abdominals and back muscles to push the pedals. Perfect for core training! In addition, you get the extra benefit of a cardio workout, which helps reduce belly fat.

A spinning class at a gym uses a stationary bike with a 40-pound wheel that allows you to increase and decrease the tension during the class. A spinning class burns more than 500 calories and takes biking to a whole new level. Try it; I know you'll like it!

Plank It

The plank exercise is one of the best core strengthening exercises. The plank position requires you to pull in your abs while you stay lifted in a push-up position with your glutes squeezed together and your back straight.

The plank exercise energizes your entire body. It's used in yoga and Pilates. So next time you're short on time, roll out of bed, drop down to the floor, and plank it!

Lengthen It

Any exercise that lengthens your core engages the muscles through stretching. Yoga and Pilates exercises use extending and lengthening exercises to help you achieve core definition.

Dancers always tend to look long and lean because they have great posture. They achieve this by having strong abdominal and back muscles. It all works hand in hand — strong abs, strong back, and good posture. It's all good!

Suck It In

In many cases, people just aren't in the habit of pulling in their tummies and sucking it in! To suck in your stomach, pretend you're tightening a belt around your waist as you're standing or sitting tall throughout the day. This technique gives you a visual reminder and helps you keep your stomach muscles tight and taut instead of letting them go slack!

Twist It

Twisting your core helps define your waist by working the *obliques* (muscles that run along the waist). The bicycle crunch is very effective for working this area. Any exercise that twists your upper body requires strong abs and back muscles.

Sports that use a twisting motion include golf and baseball. In both of them, you have to twist to hit the ball. Both sports engage the core and help develop the kind of strength you need to be a good player. Think Tiger Woods!

Ten Household Items You Can Use to Help Improve Core Strength

* * *

In This Chapter

▶ Being spontaneous with your core exercises

▶ Exercising with everyday items

* * *

You already know exercise is important, but it's also extremely helpful to do a little bit each day. Why? Because frequent exercise, even in small amounts, provides several crucial benefits:

- ✔ **Maintains your fitness level:** Even when you're short on time or you missed your workout, performing calisthenics or a few simple exercises throughout the day helps maintain your fitness level that you've worked so hard to achieve.

- ✔ **Energizes you:** When you need an energy boost and there's no coffee or chocolate in sight, try a jumping jack or two to get oxygen to your brain. You'll feel great, and you'll skip the calories!

✔ **Relieves minor aches and pains:** Exercise relieves the stress created by inactivity or repetitive motions by increasing your circulation and keeping oxygen flowing to sore muscles.

So any time can be the right time to exercise when you're at home. And believe it or not, your home is full of core-strengthening aids. The rest of this bonus excerpt points out common items you can use in your fitness routine. Now you *really* have no excuse not to stretch! And if you want more ways to strengthen your middle, pick up a copy of *Core Strength For Dummies,* available at a bookstore near you or by going to www.dummies.com!

A Chair from Your Kitchen

Sitting in a chair too long and too often doesn't loosen and relax your muscles; it actually shortens certain muscles, such as your hamstrings, hip flexors, and calves. Nevertheless, a chair can be a very useful and effective prop for exercising. And I bet you have a chair in just about every room of the house.

A basic chair exercise is the seated sit-up. To do this exercise, sit in a chair and extend your arms out in front of you. Now rise to a standing position. Notice how you're forced to use your core. Pause for a moment before sitting back down in the chair. Repeat 10 to 15 times.

Be careful, especially at work, that you don't use a chair with wheels. You can use any type of chair, as long as it's sturdy and stable.

A Beam or Rafter in Your House

Just like in the movie *Rocky,* you can hang from an open beam in your house or garage to do a pull-up. At first you'll probably only be able to hold yourself up for a few seconds, but as your grip gets stronger, you'll be able to chin up or pull yourself up to really feel the strength in your core increasing.

 If you're having trouble with this exercise, put a chair underneath the beam to help you reach it and grab on.

Your Coffee Table in the Living Room

Although you may think of your coffee table as being a good place to rest your coffee, this versatile piece of furniture makes for a great piece of exercise equipment:

- ✔ It's strong and usually made of wood, so you can do dips off of it without being afraid that it will break under your weight.

- ✔ It's off the floor, which makes it easier to get into a lot of different positions.

- ✔ It's in hotel rooms, so even when you travel, you can get a core workout!

Your Desk in Your Home Office

Your desk at home can be an excellent prop for exercising. When you need to take a break from sitting in front of the computer, you don't have to go very far to move some different muscles. Here's how to do deep lunges, using your desk for support:

1. **Stand in front of your desk and place both hands on top, making sure you're an arm's length away from it.**

2. **Lean forward into a lunge position so your right knee bends and your left leg is extended behind you.**

3. **Drop your left knee slowly to the floor as you tighten your stomach muscles to hold your body weight stable.**

4. **Inhale deeply as you press back up to a standing position, using your abs and back to keep you standing tall.**

5. **Repeat the core strengthener with the left leg.**

 If you don't have a desk handy, you can do this exercise using your dining room table or a hip-high windowsill.

A Doorway in Your Bathroom

A doorway is a great exercise prop because it's both stable and large enough to have many different applications.

Try this shoulder stretch using a doorjamb:

1. **Grab onto the molding over the top of the door with your fingertips.**

2. **Bend your knees slightly, but keep your feet on the floor until you feel a stretch in your abdominals and back muscles.**

3. **Grab onto the sides of the doorway and bend forward as if you were going to touch your toes, but keep your bend at waist level and even with your arms.**

If you're not tall enough to reach the top of the door, you can use a stepstool.

Water Jugs in Your Kitchen

Okay, now I know I'm a total nerd because I find myself doing this all the time when I refill the water machine. But those 1- to 2-gallon jugs with the handles make for a good piece of resistance equipment, don't they?

You can curl (and press, if you're really feeling energetic) your water jugs (or old milk jugs filled with water) to give your biceps a workout, as well as tone your core as you transition the movement through it. Adding weight to your core allows you to tighten this area while you maintain proper posture and focus on the individual muscles you're working.

A Towel in Your Bathroom

For core stretching, nothing beats a good, old-fashioned bath towel or smaller hand towel to help you achieve the stretch. It doesn't matter whether you're attempting a stretch for the upper or the lower body; using a towel to increase your reach makes the stretch more comfortable.

The Steps in Your House

Every time you walk up and down the steps, guess what you're working? Yep, your butt — but also your abs, hips, back, and core! I live in a three-story home, and I'm convinced I don't have to do anything else but walk up and down the stairs about 50 times a day to stay fit. Now try carrying laundry and kids up and down, too, and you'll see what I mean. If you have stairs in your house, use them! When you're done, stretch out your feet and legs with the following exercise:

1. **Stand on the bottom step with only the ball of your right foot pressed down as your left foot remains beside it. Inhale deeply.**

   Make sure you hold on to a railing or something stable to prevent you from falling.

2. **As you exhale, slowly lower your heel until you feel a comfortable stretch in your calf.**

3. **Hold the stretch for 10 to 15 seconds.**

4. **Try to gently drop your heel a little lower until you feel a deeper stretch in your calf.**

5. **Repeat the stretch on your other leg.**

An excellent variation to help you stretch your calf more deeply is to slightly bend the knee of the leg you're stretching. You should feel a difference at the base of your calf.

A Wall in Your House

You can use a wall to support any stretch. It's smooth and wide and (I know this sounds a little obvious) adjacent to the floor. It's precisely because a wall is adjacent to the floor that you have two firm, stable sources of support.

You can do push-ups using the wall instead of your coffee table. The exercise is easier when you use the wall, but it's just as effective at toning your core, and it's especially good for strengthening your back.

When you're done with your push-up, turn around and put your back flat against the wall and bend forward from your hips to let your head and arms and everything else hang out. If you can't place your palms on the floor (and face it, not many of us can), rest your hands on your shins for support. This is a great back and core strengthener.

A Book Lying on Your Nightstand

Sit on a big book to lift your hips off the floor just enough to take away some of the stress and strain of a tight lower back. When you don't feel that strain anymore, you can stretch forward to grasp your toes and focus on pulling your belly button to your spine without rounding your back.

When you do sitting exercises, try sitting on a book. You should notice how much easier it is to keep your back straight and your stomach sucked in!

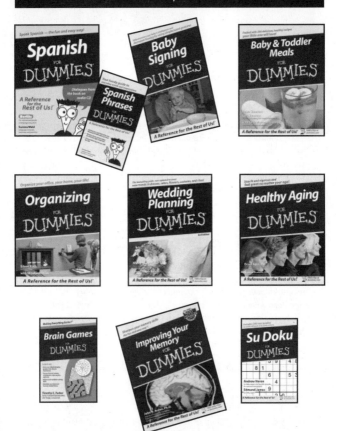

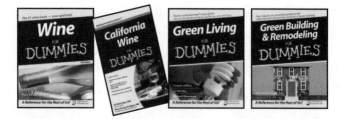

With more than 1,400 titles to choose from, we've got a Dummies book for wherever you are in life!

Business/Personal Finance & Investment

High-Powered Investing All-in-One For Dummies	9780470186268	$29.99
Investing For Dummies, 5th Edition	9780470289655	$21.99
Living Well in a Down Economy For Dummies	9780470401170	$14.99
Managing Your Money All-in-One For Dummies	9780470345467	$29.99
Personal Finance Workbook For Dummies	9780470099339	$19.99
Taxes 2009 For Dummies (January 2009)	9780470249512	$17.99

Crafts & Hobbies

California Wine For Dummies (May 2009)	9780470376072	$16.99
Canning & Preserving For Dummies	9780764524714	$16.99
Jewelry & Beading Designs For Dummies	9780470291122	$19.99
Knitting For Dummies, 2nd Edition	9780470287477	$21.99
Quilting For Dummies, 2nd Edition	9780764597992	$21.99
Watercolor Painting For Dummies	9780470182314	$24.99

Fitness & Diet

Dieting For Dummies, 2nd Edition	9780764541490	$21.99
Low-Calorie Dieting For Dummies	9780764599057	$21.99
Nutrition For Dummies, 4th Edition	9780471798682	$21.99
Exercise Balls For Dummies	9780764556234	$21.99
Fitness For Dummies, 3rd Edition	9780764578519	$21.99
Stretching For Dummies	9780470067413	$16.99

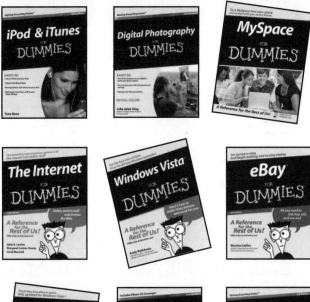
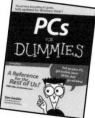
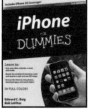
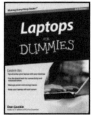